"They" Lived At Our House

Coping With Alzheimer's

Stephanie Heavey

THEY LIVED AT OUR HOUSE

The stories related in this book are those of one couple's journey through the unknown that characterizes the life of a person with Alzheimer's Disease and its effects on his or her family.

Many people with various forms of dementia or Alzheimer's Disease have problems similar to those described in this book. This book is not in any way intended to be a substitute for competent medical diagnosis, counseling or treatment. The publication of this book does not constitute the practice of medicine nor does it attempt to replace your physician.

Copyright © 2018 Stephanie Heavey

All rights reserved.

ISBN: 9781974034185
IS

This book is dedicated

to all those who are

living with dementia

in any form

and to those

who care for them

with loving hearts.

May God

wrap

His Arms

around You.

In Loving Memory of Jack Heavey

1929 - 2006

CONTENTS

Prologue		vii
Chapter One	1966	1
Chapter Two	2000	4
Chapter Three	2001	9
Chapter Four	2002	14
Chapter Five	2003	20
Chapter Six	2004	29
Chapter Seven	2005	61
Chapter Eight	2006	128
Epilogue		213
Notes		215

THEY LIVED AT OUR HOUSE

Prologue

How does it begin? When? It is like looking at an intriguing 1,000-piece puzzle, full and complete, delighting all who look at it. A piece pops out and falls to the floor. After awhile another falls out. Then another. The pieces begin to fall faster, taking others with them. Soon the subject of the picture is no longer discernible.

And that, to me, is Alzheimer's Disease.

In the early stages, there is little to distinguish Alzheimer's Disease from what one perceives as the little foibles of aging. A slowing of thoughts, forgetting a name here and there, a bit of irritation, some loss of sense of humor. When I first began to suspect that these changes in my husband Jack were more than senior moments, I read books, magazines, newspaper articles, the internet. Everything was read eagerly in hope of finding another clue to prove, or better yet, disprove my sinking realizations.

There was nothing I found that gave concrete examples of the changes that occur in the early stages of Alzheimer's. The closest I came was reading about a woman who said she realized her husband's forgetfulness was more than ordinary when he could not remember different brews of beer while tending bar at a fundraiser, something he had been doing for years. Every time I read about the keys in the sugar bowl or the forgetting of the grandchildren's names, or not remembering how to get back home, I grew more frustrated. What about way before that? How does it start?

What is the difference between an ordinary memory lapse and one that indicates Alzheimer's? The events that troubled me were, at first, few and far between. One would occur and unsettle me. Then life would go on day by day and I would decide that I was making mountains out of molehills. Then something unusual would occur again.

Journaling was begun in the hope that the entries would let me see whether a pattern was developing. It would be much more accurate than relying on memory for exactly when, where, and what happened, especially if these occurrences were the result of a medical condition. This book is the result of that journal. It is only my experience with Alzheimer's as it affected the love of my life, my husband Jack.

Jack was a quiet man. A graphic artist who was intelligent and very creative, but also unobtrusive. As such, he probably wouldn't approve of this book. However, if one victim of AD is helped because a caregiver finds something in this book to make life easier for that person, if one caregiver is helped because this book gives him or her a slightly better understanding of what is happening, then my goal will be achieved. And of that, my compassionate Jack would approve.

CHAPTER ONE

Snow fell in large soft flakes on the icy waters of Lake Michigan, on the curves of Lake Shore Drive, on the observation decks of the Hancock and Prudential Buildings, on Chicago's City Hall and all the sentinels along Michigan Avenue. It fell quietly on the Eisenhower Expressway as it shot cars like arrows straight out into the silent streets of the western suburbs.

We were in one of those cars that frigid January night in 1966. The soft quiet music of Franklyn MacCormack's late night radio show muffled the crunch of the tires on the accumulating snow.

Jack was preoccupied all evening. From the time he picked me up, he was unusually quiet. About what was he thinking? We saw a movie and stopped at a little café on Rush Street for tea and biscuits. He barely sipped his coffee and nibbled at a biscuit. His mind was struggling with something.

We exited the expressway and drove slowly along the snow-packed streets of Oak Park, his blue eyes gazing steadily at the road, but his brow betraying an inner turmoil. He slowed the car and parked it along a seldom trafficked side street. For a few moments all was still and quiet while we watched snowflakes hide the view through the windshield.

Jack turned in his seat to face me and I turned toward him. Hesitantly, he began to say that there was something I needed to know about him. We had worked together in the same medical building for four years, but until three weeks ago, all our contact with each other had been strictly professional.

He asked me if I knew how old he was. I was twenty-two and knew he was in his thirties. If I guessed older than he was, it would hurt his feelings which I couldn't bear to do; younger would make it harder for him to tell me he was older. It didn't matter to me but I could see that it mattered to him. I guessed thirty-two. He reluctantly corrected it to thirty-six.

Hesitancy still filled his voice as he started to explain that he was diabetic and that the disease had lifelong complications. I replied that I knew about diabetes and its effect on the body from my days of researching diseases in medical literature. And I knew he was diabetic since his hospitalization the prior year. It made no difference to me. I loved him for who he was, not what he was.

His face was calm but his eyes and that little furrow in his brow told me there was still something on his mind. But what? He always seemed quiet, responsible, dependable, dedicated, with a tenacious spirit. In the past three weeks I found he was also very fun loving, humorous, compassionate. Once we began talking about more than the medical journal on which we both worked, it was easy to realize how deep a man he was in his thinking and beliefs and ideals. What else could he view as a problem?

As I gazed at him wondering what was to come, he took my hand in his. He told me how happy he had been these last three weeks. He would give me the world if he could. He loved me. And would I do him the honor of being his wife?

My heart skipped beats and my mind twirled. In these wonderful weeks, marriage had never entered my mind. I just knew I loved him and wanted to be with him.

Jack saw my hesitation and quietly said I didn't have to answer. Perhaps it was too soon. He should have waited.

But every fiber of my being disagreed. This was right. It was meant to be. And the girl who agonized over every decision to change jobs or buy a car or even what to wear, gave an unequivocal 'Yes!' And changed her entire life in that second.

As we melted into each other's arms, the Buick was like a reverse snow globe: warm and snug inside while snow fell all around outside. Like a snow globe, life had been turned upside down in the most wonderful way.

Suddenly, Jack was hungry. We drove the unplowed streets of several suburbs trying to find a coffee shop that was open at three in the morning. Not an easy task in 1966. As I sat in the booth gazing at the snow flakes still falling outside the window, I wondered where the future would take us. In how many coffee shop booths would we sit over how many years? The future spread itself out before us, unknown and tantalizing.

Thirty-five years later, the snow would fall again. Only this time it would be the plaque of Alzheimer's Disease falling on the mind of Jack and destroying every brain cell it touched. And once again life would be turned upside down.

◊◊◊◊◊◊◊◊◊◊

CHAPTER TWO

Saturday, January 1, 2000

The millennium has arrived. And the world has survived. All the precautionary measures people took "just in case" were mostly for naught. So we are all sitting with full tanks of gas in our vehicles, extra provisions in our basements and extra cash in our wallets.

Even without the "what if all the computers fail when the clock strikes midnight" angst, the dawn of a new millennium, not just another year or another century, merits thoughts of the unknown future. What will it be like? What will happen? Will times be better or worse?

There are bound to be changes for Jack and me. After all, he is seventy - a whole new decade of life. After our engagement, when I used to read the obituaries of the doctors who died from diabetic complications, hoping to get an idea of how many years we might have together, the magic number seemed to be seventy. And now we are there. Thankfully, Jack has not had any major complications. All he has had is minor diabetic retinopathy in his eyes which was resolved with a laser.

However, there is one thing that is bothering me. There have been little signs of change that seem unusual. They are few and far between. I don't know if I am reading more into them than is there. Perhaps writing things down when they happen will give me a better perspective in the long run. Is there a pattern? Or is it just natural aging?

I seem to be losing my best friend. Jack is irritable much more frequently. And I am at a loss to know why. I find myself wondering if there is something I said or did or didn't do that is bothering him. In the past, we would let each other know if something was annoying us. If I ask now, it just increases the irritation. Does he sense a change but doesn't know why, which is what really irritates him?

Like many couples married for a long time, Jack and I can often finish each other's sentences, read each other's thoughts. We can observe a situation, look at each other and know what the other is thinking without saying a word.

"Did you take..."
"Yeah, I did."
"I thought you were going to..."
"I know but instead I decided to..."
"Figured you would."

Now Jack doesn't seem to pick up on my cues.

"Oh, honey, look at that!"
No response.
"Doesn't that remind you of our trip to New Orleans?"
Puzzled look.
"Remember the trip to the bayous and how hot it was?"
Still puzzled.
"Remember the maître d' who stood so still we thought he was a cardboard cutout?"
No light bulbs going off.
"Remember it was the first time I flew. You were eager to give me that experience. I thought the takeoff from O'Hare was terrific. Later, you mentioned to me that the plane had eaten up too much runway and you thought we might crash before we were airborne." Nothing.

For the most part, though, he can still regale family and friends with all those wonderful stories of our trips, his service in Korea, his career experiences. Just sometimes, he draws a blank.

I've begun to read articles on aging and dementia. So far, none of them have given me a clue as to why these changes are occurring. Does it have a psychological origin or a physical one?

THEY LIVED AT OUR HOUSE

Wednesday, March 15, 2000

Jack received in the mail an offer promoting a trip to Hawaii for a fantastic price. He seemed enthusiastic. It had been his plan to honeymoon in Hawaii. An idea that was put on hold for financial reasons. Over the years, however, we would talk about it, but the timing never seemed right.

Sitting at the sewing machine attaching eyelet to a hundred little doll dresses, the idea took root in my mind. This is my twelfth year in the business designing and producing specialty clothing for the vastly popular 18-inch dolls. This will be an easy year. There are no plans to expand into more stores or add shows to our already busy fall calendar. The stores and shows through which we sell the doll clothes are the most profitable. We are at a point where we could vacation somewhere like Hawaii.

At lunch I asked Jack if he was seriously thinking about the trip. In response he began mentioning minor ailments that are bothering him. He never answered the question directly.

Recently, he has become more concerned with his health and how he is feeling from day to day. Little things like an upset stomach will concern him greatly. In the past, he wouldn't give it a second thought. Now he reminds me of his mom who obsessed over every minor ailment, partly because she had little to fill her days and partly because her parents had died at young ages and she thought she would do the same.

Tuesday, May 30, 2000

Another troubling sign. Jack has always had a prodigious knowledge of famous people: politicians, movie stars, artists, the Fortune 500. Fiction holds no interest for him. Biographies and autobiographies are his delight. He has been a prize asset on any Trivial Pursuit team. Suddenly, he is having great difficulty remembering names. All the time. Not just once in a while. He remembers facts but the names are elusive.

And so we play twenty questions. It's not an even match because my knowledge is so much more limited than his.

I'm sitting at the sewing machine working on doll clothes. Jack appears in the doorway to the sewing room.

"Come and see Larry King. He has that guy on."

"What guy?"

"You know, the one who used to be president."

"Bush?"

"No."

"Well, it can't be Reagan. Ford?"

"No! You know, the one who's all over."

"They're all going about giving speeches."

"No, the one who's actually doing some good."

"You mean Jimmy Carter?"

"Yes. That's the one."

He smiles in great satisfaction, turns around and walks back to the family room.

Tuesday, November 28, 2000

Jack had a snow shovel that he purchased from a catalog years ago and assembled. It was a handy shovel with a diagonal front that pushed snow off to the edge of the pavement. The handle finally broke last year and he was dismayed. I found one in a catalog this year and gave it to him for his birthday on the 22nd.

He was in the basement all afternoon. When I went down to let him know dinner was ready, I found him trying to put the shovel together. The blade was on wrong. He was very upset. "I can't figure this out. **They** wrote the instructions all wrong. The diagram isn't right. I've put this blade on and off five times and nothing works. I'd like to see **them** put a hundred of these things together. Then maybe **they** would think before putting the directions together."

Hoping to help, and looking at the directions, I suggested that the blade should be turned around on the handle. Bad move. It only provoked more impatience. "You think you can do this? Okay, you try it. I've been working on this all afternoon but if you think you can do it in five minutes, go ahead."

In the past, Jack would be eager to be done with dinner and tackle the project again. He did not do so tonight. Not a good sign.

◊◊◊◊◊◊◊◊◊◊

CHAPTER THREE

Monday, January 1, 2001
Just a few minutes to journal before Jack's sister LaVerne arrives for dinner. Every year when her sister, Lee, goes to visit her daughter for the holidays, LaVerne celebrates with us. She hates it when her sister is not near and blames the daughter. No matter how many times we talk about Lee wanting to see her daughter and her grandchildren, LaVerne will not hear of it. She cannot understand why her sister should leave her alone and go off by herself. More and more she is attaching herself to Lee and becoming dependent on her.

Frequently, LaVerne will misplace things or leave them behind. Then she gets into a panic when she cannot find what is lost or misplaced. Their tour in Europe last year was not an easy trip. Lee realized that she had to be alert for both of them. She and I have wondered whether LaVerne has Alzheimer's.

As far as Jack is concerned, the holidays were without incident. The two of us and our daughter, Tricia, had a most memorable Christmas. Jack has always been known to find the most thoughtful and unusual gifts. This year was no exception. We had fun-filled holidays with all the family.

Tuesday, April 24, 2001
Nothing major has gone on in the past few months to raise concern about Jack's mental abilities. Until today.

Jack bought a garden tool holder that will keep rakes and shovels and brooms together in a small space. It's a wooden square divided into sections so that each handle can be inserted separately from the others, making it easy to get tools in and out.

He spent the whole day trying to put it together. At the end of the day, all he had was a pile of wooden pieces. Once again, he could not make sense of the directions and was upset because **they** didn't know how to write instructions and he would like to see **them** put one of these things together. He gathered up the pieces and dumped them into an empty box.

That's not like Jack. In thirty-five years, he has never walked away from a project, difficult or not. Never.

Saturday, July 21, 2001

Today, Jack and I and Tricia, drove to my cousin's Annual Family Reunion. Tom has an open backyard which flows into his neighbors' yards. Everywhere there is a riot of brilliant color adorning the sweep of emerald green grass. Huge trees stand guard overhead and shade the deck and gazebo. All is bathed in the sunny warmth of a midwestern July.

My siblings and their spouses were there, as were the nieces and their children. The cousins from Bloomington drove up. For many years our lives took all of us in different directions and we saw each other infrequently. These annual reunions are cherished and eagerly anticipated.

Each year, there is much catching up to do, much food, much laughter and fun. Today was no exception. The three of us left the reunion in a happy, contented mood.

Which lasted until we neared the Roosevelt Road exit on Route 355. The sun was just slipping behind the trees to the west when traffic ground to a halt. Beyond the parking lot of cars in front of us, we could see the flashing red and blue lights of ambulances and police cars. Two police cars cordoned off the expressway and all cars were required to exit.

We found ourselves being carried along in a mass of vehicles heading east on Roosevelt Road. Jack was upset and concerned. "Where are we going?" It was an astonishing remark.

He sounded lost. Yet this area was part of his "old stomping grounds." As a kid he used to ride his bike down Roosevelt Road to its western end. The first forty-two years of his life had been lived in the western suburbs straddling Roosevelt Road.

It was unsettling to realize that he was not sure which roads would get us home. Together we had only lived in the western suburbs for six years before moving northwest of Chicago. My knowledge of the area is quite small compared to his. Gradually I recognized exactly where we were and steered us to Route 83 heading north. It was only when we were about five miles from home that Jack visibly relaxed because the surroundings were now familiar to him.

I cannot relax. My mind is in turmoil. This is *not* normal aging. The depth of confusion is just too great to be a senior moment. Dear Lord, what is happening?

Tuesday, September 11, 2001

A day never to be forgotten. Jack went to the bank. I was in the kitchen cleaning up after breakfast. LaVerne called. "Do you have the TV on? Turn it on! I can't believe what's happening!" I turned on the TV just in time to see the plane crash into the second World Trade Tower. Then to hear that the Pentagon had also been hit and that another plane was hijacked somewhere in Pennsylvania. Never have I felt so vulnerable. When Jack came home, we both sat in the family room glued to the TV and all the events unfolding. It was unreal to see two skyscrapers fall to the ground like so much sand.

With all air travel grounded for a few days, a concern is that our impending trip to Las Vegas for the International Sewing Convention might be canceled. Did we even want to fly with such uncertainty? I feel that once the planes are back in the air again, it will probably be the safest time to travel because everyone will be hyper-vigilant.

Thursday, September 27 - Wednesday, October 3, 2001

Two weeks have passed and we are in Las Vegas which had become a ghost town while all the planes were grounded. So many people are afraid to fly. The tourist business, the life blood of Vegas, is suffering. The convention itself is noticeably lacking in attendance and rather somber. All the talk revolves around people who had worked in the Trade Towers: relatives, friends or business acquaintances of the exhibitors.

Throughout the week, while Jack has kept the hectic pace, I can see that it is tiring for him, not physically, but mentally. So much happening so fast. So much to see and hear and absorb. He looks to me to make all the reservations and decisions. How totally different from our earlier trips, when he would make all the arrangements and then tell me what he had planned.

On October 1st, our 35th Wedding Anniversary, we took a gondola ride down the lovely canal at the Venetian Hotel. The gondolier tried to get a romantic response out of Jack but met failure. Jack didn't seem to understand what was being asked. Another unsettling moment. In the past, he would have had his arm around me and been smiling.

Afterward, we walked through Bellagio and stopped outside to watch the dancing waters. It was a beautiful night with a full moon rising just above the replica of the Eiffel Tower at the hotel Paris across the street and a warm desert breeze gently touching one's cheek. As the waters cascaded to the music of *Time to Say Goodbye,* I held Jack's hand. The thought occurred that in the past several years, I'd been losing Jack very slowly but surely. Had the time to say goodbye already begun?

Saturday, November 10, 2001

Jack and his alarm clock are not on friendly terms. He sets it at night if we need to get up at a specific time. In the morning, the alarm never sounds. And the switch is off. He is frustrated and has cautioned me "not to touch it because it will really be messed up." From time to time he comments that other clocks aren't working right.

Thursday, December 6, 2001
    Jack is having trouble remembering the craft show schedules this year even though I gave him a copy and we've talked about them several times. Today, at lunch, I said,
    "We'll have to leave here on Saturday about 6 a.m. so we can be there by 7 a.m. to set up."
    "Be where?"
    "At the Hinsdale House."
    "You never told me about that one."
    "I did when we talked about all the shows."
    "You never mentioned that one."
    "It's on the list. I gave you a copy."
    "I never saw it. You didn't give me one."
    "I put it on your drawing board."
    "I don't have it. You think you gave it to me but you didn't. Lately, you've been doing this more and more. What's going on?"
    What is going on???

CHAPTER FOUR

Tuesday, January 1, 2002
    Two years have gone by since I began journaling with the intent of seeing whether my concerns about Jack are following a pattern or are just sporadic. There are small glitches that occur on a regular basis So far, the troubling occurrences are widely spaced.
    However, his inability to remember the names of famous people has become entrenched. The names of places are also becoming difficult to remember. He has started to complain that he is having a hard time finding things because **they** misplaced it, **they** moved it, etc.

Tuesday, February 12, 2002
    Jack ordered a thirty-one slot bill organizer for mail. He has always paid every bill ten days before the due date without fail. He said this separator will be a big help because "**they** are sending so much mail, it is hard keeping track of it." Tonight he set it up and put each bill in the slot for the day which is ten days prior to when the bill is due.

Wednesday, April 10, 2002
    Periodically, Jack is having trouble with buttons, dials and switches on clocks, radios, his camera. Every so often, he will be stymied about how to operate them. Appliances and gadgets he has used for many years will suddenly seem foreign to him. In frustration he will often comment that **they** should try operating this or **they** don't know how to design something. This is quite

noticeable when he gets in the car and presses a button that opens a window instead of the door or pops the trunk. He explains it away by saying, "It isn't easy when you are driving two cars."

Fortunately, his driving skills are as sharp as ever. He keeps the posted speed, practices all the rules of the road and is very aware of what all the other drivers on the road are doing. I feel comfortable riding with him.

Saturday, July 27, 2002

Today my nieces hosted a combination 40th Wedding Anniversary/70th Birthday Party for their mom and dad. The 28th will be their folks' 40th Wedding Anniversary and the 29th will be their dad's 70th birthday. We started off bright and early with the 40/70 box secure in the trunk. It has been fun the past few weeks finding items that totaled either forty or seventy - a box of 40 envelopes, 70 sheets of paper toweling, 70 screws in a jar, a 40-watt light bulb, a photo of a 40-mile an hour speed limit sign, etc.

The trip was uneventful until we reached Indiana. Instead of turning right on the feeder road, Jack turned left. The road was closed a half mile up for road construction and we had to detour which took us on a back road that meandered this way and that until we finally reached Route 30. We lost all the lead time we had and the unknown detour over gravelly roads rattled both the car and our nerves.

The day itself was warm, windy and wonderful. Another opportunity to be with siblings, extended family and friends, some of whom we hadn't seen since the last family wedding. Over the years my sister has taken upon herself the joyful task of keeping in touch with all the far flung relatives. Today was the day when we were all together celebrating her anniversary because of her dedication. It was a day filled with reminiscing and laughter and nostalgia for the years when we were growing up together.

As we waved our goodbyes pulling out of the driveway, and settled in for the long drive home, Jack said he was not going back the way we came. He was going to use Route 41 to 30 west. In the past he avoided both roads because they are stoplight-laden commercial thoroughfares, overburdened with local traffic. Thirty-five years is ample time to learn when not to say anything and so I didn't. Not when we passed Route 41. Not when we passed the feeder road. Not when we ended up in the same construction mess we had been in earlier in the day.

My voice may have been silent, but my mind was not. Thoughts were crashing into each other. This was not like Jack. He didn't even realize that he had crossed over Route 41 instead of turning on to it. He didn't seem to recognize that he wasn't on the feeder road until we came to the construction detour. He was at a loss to understand why he was back in the same mess we had been in earlier. The frustration coming from the driver's seat was palpable. Tricia and I said nothing which helped the moment to pass.

The changes in her dad's behavior and actions have puzzled Tricia. She has great empathy for people and can sense when someone is unhappy or ill sooner than most people. For her, things are black and white. Nuances in attitude and behavior sometimes elude her. So these sporadic changes confuse her, as they do me. She wants to deal with them on the surface, each one as it comes. I have been explaining to her that there could be a problem that is causing all of these unusual incidents. It is difficult for her to accept that possibility.

Tuesday, October 1, 2002
Today was our 36th Wedding Anniversary. LaVerne and Lee were invited to join us for dinner.

THEY LIVED AT OUR HOUSE

LaVerne loves to eat in restaurants. She is not a hearty eater. But she loves all kinds of food and dishes and always seasons our conversations with descriptions of her most recent dining experiences. While Jack will only have fruit or sherbet for dessert, his sisters love desserts, especially chocolate ones. LaVerne enjoys all the different dishes she is served as the prelude to dessert. Her sister would gladly skip dinner and go directly to dessert.

Jack intended to treat his sisters to dinner at our favorite restaurant: salad and steak or fish topped off by the dessert sampler which has scrumptious portions of cheesecake, torte, pie, fruit, tiramisu. However, the best laid plans of mice and men...

As soon as the five of us were seated and LaVerne opened her menu, her penny-pinching instincts surfaced. Only this time she was counting her brother's pennies and not her own. She promptly said she wasn't hungry and began looking for the least expensive dish on the menu. Lee had her eye on a pecan-crusted walleye fillet with rice and salad. But as soon as she realized what LaVerne was doing, she decided to follow suit. LaVerne was adamant in her choice and grew testy when I tried to change her mind. She declared that the prices were outrageous (they are not) and she was not going to have her brother pay that kind of money.

Jack's happy outlook changed when he realized what was going on. After all, it was our anniversary. He had wanted to host this celebration and LaVerne was sabotaging it. She claimed that she could not eat another thing so the dessert sampler would be a waste. Trying to salvage some of the evening, I suggested going back to our house for coffee and a cake that I had on hand. To Jack's irritation, LaVerne's appetite was totally revitalized by the time the cake and ice cream were served.

Afterward, Jack gave me a beautifully wrapped box. Within was an absolutely exquisite silver bracelet. Immediately, I tried it on. It is too large for my wrist. Jack said we would take it to the jeweler and have it resized. There is a small section that could be removed without changing the design of the bracelet.

    LaVerne glowered. "Take it and get your money back. Where would you wear something so nice, anyway?"

    "LaVerne! It's our anniversary. It's a gift from Jack."

    "It's ridiculous. Why keep something you will never use?"

    Because Jack gave it to me. I will wear it. I never return anything he has given me. I know how much thought he puts into each gift. His thought and effort in selecting an item are as much a gift to me as is the item itself. His actions and his gifts have always been signs of his love and caring.

    But the damage was done and the evening ended on a strained note. Recently, I have noticed that when LaVerne and Jack are together, there is tension in the air. Neither one seems to understand what the other is doing or saying and there is conflict. LaVerne has always spoken in a know-it-all tone. For the most part, Jack would ignore what she said and move on. Lately, he will no longer do that. He will stand firm in his opinion and will not back down. Both seem to have a need to be the one who is right. Is it becoming necessary to be right to invalidate the suspicion that something is wrong with one's memory?

Tuesday, December 10, 2002

    At last, the final doll show of the holiday season is over. The pressure is off, at least for another year. Every week there is a time crunch to sew the doll costumes, do the handwork, tag them, and pack the Polish luggage (large heavyweight shopping bags) and plastic containers with the dolls, costumes, hooks, accessories, signage, order forms and other show necessities. The Polish luggage is efficient. The dresses sit lightly in the bags and don't crush. I can carry three bags in each hand into and out of a show venue which makes setup and takedown easier. And the bags can be lined up on the back seat of the Chevy holding more inventory in the space than the plastic containers.

Jack and I have been a team doing the shows for the past fifteen years. I supply the inventory. He makes the displays and packs everything into the vehicle. He has been a master at making the maximum use of space. Until now. This year it has been a struggle. For the first time he has needed help in getting everything into the trunk. He has insisted that I have more inventory than in previous years. I've tried to fit more into the back seat so there is less to put into the trunk. Even so, fitting everything into the trunk is still difficult for him.

The first show we did, I noticed that Jack had trouble setting up the displays, especially the lighting. By the end of the day, he was exhausted. For the remainder of the season, Tricia has accompanied us. She was a big help in bringing everything into the building while I set up the back displays and the lighting. After the booth was complete, Jack returned home to rest and she worked with me. Jack would return about an hour before the show ended to do takedown.

Years ago, when we did the first few shows, Jack laughed. He said it was like the circus. At six in the morning, there was a totally empty auditorium, cafeteria, or gymnasium. In two or three hours, the space was converted into a kaleidoscope of color and texture. At the end of the day, within an hour, the venue was empty with no clue that a show had ever been there.

Once again, the signs I see appear to be more than just natural aging. I do know that I will curtail the shows I do next fall to the most profitable ones. No profit is worth the toll it is taking on Jack.

◊◊◊◊◊◊◊◊◊

CHAPTER FIVE

Wednesday, January 1, 2003
Three years and I still don't know exactly what is causing these unpredictable changes in Jack. Daily life continues, but there is always this unsettling feeling just under the surface. It is an unspoken tension that permeates each day. It ebbs. As I begin to relax, another perplexing situation occurs.

Slowly, Jack is having trouble remembering nouns. Of great significance, he has started to use the word "shot" to indicate testing his blood glucose as well as taking a dose of insulin. For the past forty years, he has always checked his blood glucose and administered his insulin independently. He is adamant that it will continue that way. But now when I ask him if he took a blood glucose reading, he will say he took a "shot." If I ask him whether or not he took insulin, he will say he took a "shot". I am at a loss to know exactly what he did. Missing readings wouldn't be the ideal, but overdosing on insulin could be fatal.

Throughout our married life, when Jack's behavior seemed odd or unnatural for him, I would suspect a hypoglycemic (low blood sugar) episode and suggest he test his blood glucose level which would always be low. He would drink a glass of orange juice and within twenty minutes, everything would be normal.

Lately, the tests do not always show a low level of glucose. Could these odd episodes be due to diabetic gastric neuropathy or insulin resistance? Could each hypoglycemic episode have a cumulative effect on brain function? I've been researching it on the internet.

As long-term type one diabetics age, neuropathy causes a loss of the sensitivity which at a younger age enables them to be aware of the first signs of hypoglycemia. As a result, the low glucose level isn't treated promptly, continues to drop, and then creates a very noticeable decline in one's mental activity and consciousness.

Wednesday, February 12, 2003

The budget book has become a source of aggravation for both of us. Being the creature of habit that he is, for the past thirty-six years, Jack has fastidiously recorded every expense we have incurred in his budget book. It is a binder full of loose-leaf pages with columns for food, medicine, utilities, clothing, household expenses, etc., as well as one for miscellaneous expenses. At the end of each month, I tally up the columns to see what was spent in each category. The column totals are then added up to see what was spent that month.

It has been a good system in that we both are aware of how much is being spent each month and on what. Until now.

Tonight I finished adding up the totals for the last several months. I always get behind in the fall because of the doll shows and accelerated production. I gave the book back to Jack and began working on the business income taxes. Five minutes later, Jack came and put the book on my desk.

"You didn't add these columns right."

I looked everything over and said, "It looks okay to me."

"No, it isn't. You didn't add the credit card payment into the total."

"I never do that since every credit card purchase is already listed in a specific column. If I added it into the monthly total, it would show that we spent more than we actually did. It would be adding the same amount in twice."

"You never have done that? Then all the totals are wrong!"

"No, Jack. They are okay."

"But you didn't add the credit card payment in!"

"Because each amount on the credit card statement has already been written in a specific column."

"But the amount isn't added into the total."

"Because the smaller amounts that make up the total on the credit card statement are already added in to different columns."

"But it's not in the total and it should be."

"It is part of the total because the smaller amounts are already in each column."

"But it's not in the total."

Around and around we went for fifteen minutes while the level of agitation grew.

Finally, I said, "Jack, trust me. The totals are correct." It ended the disagreement. But I could see by the look on his face that Jack was still convinced the totals are wrong and that I had messed up the budget book.

It is the abstracts that mystify Jack. The whole concept of numbers and what they mean and how they interact, dates, time and the chronology of time. It pains me to see his uncertainty or outright confusion.

Saturday, March 15, 2003

The Ides of March. And I am beginning to feel like Julius Caesar waiting for the next stab of anxiety. According to Jack, his clocks still aren't working right. The concept of time is becoming very tenuous.

"Today is Tuesday, right?"

"Tomorrow is garbage day, right?"

Something all of us do, but not umpteen times a day, right?

Saturday, April 5, 2003

A flyer inserted with his credit card statement caused Jack much angst.

"Just look at this. After all the years with that bank, **they're** accusing me of taking advantage of them!"

He handed me the flyer. It was a marketing tool for the loan department. In bold letters and large type, it asked "Are you taking advantage of Us?" It then showed a special 3.99% apr offered to "our most valued card members."

"You aren't being accused of anything, Jack. Look, this is a special offer for valued customers, like you. They are offering people a very low annual percentage rate if you carry a balance on your card."

"Why would **they** send this to me? I always pay my bill."

"It's a mass mailing, Jack. One of these flyers goes into each envelope."

"But why would **they** send it to me?"

"Jack, it's a mass mailing. Everyone gets one with their statement."

"But I always pay on time. Something's not right."

"I'll just toss it in the wastebasket, Jack. It doesn't mean anything."

"No, let me have it. Something isn't right here."

As he left the room clutching the flyer, my heart sank. Something isn't right here. Several times now he has shown me junk mail letters. Each time he has thought that he has to respond to it, especially if his name is on it. And each time I have had to convince him that it is advertising, part of a mass mailing. And always he walks away still unsure. All this, after spending over thirty-five years working as a graphic artist in marketing and in advertising producing mass mailings.

Although I am loathe to admit it because the thought breaks my heart, more and more I *know* that all these aberrations are the result of significant dementia, most likely Alzheimer's. As I read about its progression and effects, I can think of no other disease that so cruelly robs its victims of the very attributes that define them.

Tuesday, April 29, 2003
    I am beginning to dread any advertising. Today the culprit is a newspaper ad combining a contest and coupons.
    "Look at these stupid advertising people. **They** don't know what **they** are doing. How can you mail these coupons in to enter the contest and still use them at the store?"
    I could not convince him that the coupons were not to be mailed, only used at the store. Doing so, automatically entered a person in the contest. We went round and round and round until he said,
    "Well, **they** are so very stupid **they** put in coupons that are already expired."
    I looked at the expiration dates: 5/15/03 and 6/15/03.

Sunday, June 15, 2003
    Father's Day. Tricia treated her dad to dinner. It was a very easygoing day. Jack was relaxed and enjoyed the meal. Now that the weather is warm, he has been working outside most days and benefits, both mentally and physically, from the fresh air and exercise.

Tuesday, July 15, 2003
    Jack and I went downtown to Northwestern Hospital where I had an appointment. It has been three years since we were in the Loop and on Michigan Avenue. While I was not looking forward to the medical appointment, I was looking forward to being downtown again together. Since we had met each other while working in the city, it has special memories for us.
    Jack worked in downtown Chicago from the time he was in high school until he took a position with a company in the northwestern suburbs. He loved the fast pace and action. There was always movement and noise and light and life in the city.

He knew every nook and cranny of the Loop and Michigan Avenue and the adjacent streets.

We took the Metra train, then boarded the express bus which took us to Water Tower Place. From there it was a short walk to the hospital. On the return trip, we had to walk down to Ohio Street to catch the bus heading back to the train station. That confused Jack.

"Are you sure we're going the right way?" from the guy who knew the downtown area like the back of his hand. Sure, there are a few new skyscrapers. They never mattered before. The street grid has not changed. Jack has.

Tuesday, July 29, 2003
One of my sisters called and asked if we had made plans for August 10th, my sixtieth birthday. Since we hadn't, she said that she was coming out with family and bringing dinner. All we had to do was relax.

Jack was concerned. "Where will everyone sit? How will we be able to set up for everyone?" I assured him that my sister had everything well thought out.

Tuesday, August 5, 2003
My sister called. She was not feeling well and the party was put on hold. I told her to take care of herself and forget about everything else. She was insistent that she will have this party, just not yet.

Sunday, August 10, 2003
My sixtieth birthday was a quiet day. My brother, Frank, sent a colorful bouquet of flowers from all my siblings. Jack and I attended early morning Mass and ate breakfast at a local coffee

shop afterward. Then we drove to the riverboat casino to see if sixty was a lucky year for me. It was for both of us. The day was capped off by dinner at our favorite restaurant. Thank You, God, for a beautiful, memorable birthday.

Saturday, September 20, 2003

Today was the day my family decided on as the day to celebrate my birthday. The siblings and their families attended. My sister and her daughters brought everything, food, plates, cups, flatware, etc. I didn't have to lift a finger.

The number of people present and the flurry of activity when they arrived was overwhelming for Jack. He sat quietly trying to take it all in. Once in a while he would have a short conversation with someone. Gone are the days when he and his brother-in-law would sit for hours talking and laughing about the crazy things that happened when they were in military service.

Wednesday, October 15, 2003

Tonight was D Day, or should I say AD Day. I was busily sewing away. Jack asked me how to write an amount in cursive on a check. As I quickly wrote the answer on a slip of paper, *I suddenly realized that this was exactly what I had done when Tricia was learning how to use a checkbook.* Jack was oblivious to the oddity of it all. He clutched the slip of paper, smiled, and walked out of the sewing room. And my heart shattered into a thousand pieces. I *know* he has Alzheimer's.

Thursday, October 30, 2003

Since that evening two weeks ago, every time Jack writes a check, he always writes the amount on a piece of scrap paper and asks me to okay it. He says, "sometimes the numbers don't look right." He now pays a bill as soon as it comes in. This is a good coping mechanism, since the 31-day bill holder is no longer helping him remember when to pay the bills.

Saturday, November 15, 2003
    LaVerne called tonight. Her voice was full of agitation. Every Saturday, she has gone to dinner with a friend of hers. It is the highlight of her week. She loves any opportunity to dress up and go out. The next day I am always be the recipient of a phone call describing what she wore, where they went and what delicious food was served. Tonight, her friend called her. He couldn't go out with her anymore. It was too hard. He wasn't feeling well.
    She was angry. "How can he do this to me? I've never had a man dump me! What will I do now?" I asked her why he wasn't feeling well. "He didn't say and I don't care."

Saturday, December 6, 2003
    Today was a bittersweet day for me. After fifteen years, it was the last craft show I will do selling the doll costumes. We only did three shows this year.
    Three shows were too much for Jack. He had to expend so much mental as well as physical energy trying to remember how to pack the car for every show that he was totally exhausted afterward.
    All good things must come to an end and so has this one.

Thursday, December 25, 2003
    Jack spent much time and effort this year in selecting Christmas gifts. He gave me several beautiful outfits and a gorgeous hooded leather jacket lined with faux fur. He outdid

himself. The gift I treasured most was seeing him pleased with himself because he was successful in what he set out to do.

When we were dating, I had told Jack the story of how I first learned about St. Nicholas putting candies in little kids' socks on December 6th. It had been talked about in school one December when I was in third grade. It seemed like a great thing to an 8-year-old girl. So that night I put my sock on the bedpost and went to sleep confident that I would find a bonanza of candy in the morning.

When I awoke, the sock was as flat as it had been the night before. I had not mentioned my plan to my mom or sisters. Why should I? After all, it was St. Nicholas who filled the stockings. My childish dream was to show them my good fortune in the morning.

We bought our first house in 1972, complete with wood burning fireplace in the living room. That December 6th, I was exhausted after a stressful day at work. Jack met me at the train station as always. Grateful to be home, I walked into the living room to relax for a few minutes before fixing dinner. There on the mantel was a stocking full of my favorite candy bars. St. Nicholas might have forgotten, but not Jack.

◊◊◊◊◊◊◊◊◊◊

CHAPTER SIX

Thursday, January 1, 2004
 Jack took a blood glucose reading after midnight. It was a little high after a festive dinner and a glass of wine. He insisted that he needed insulin. It was stressful convincing him that he never takes insulin at night. What a start to a Happy New Year!

Monday, January 12, 2004
 Jack kept waking up and looking at the digital clock and thinking the time was a blood glucose reading - 230, 315, 440. Could not convince him that he was looking at the digital clock and that the numbers were time and not glucose readings. At 4:40 a.m., he took a glucose reading. It was a bit high at 169 (the norm is 100 or less). However, it was not a high enough reading to warrant extra insulin. He took 15 units of insulin, anyway.
 At 8:48 a.m., he was hypoglycemic and in a semi-conscious state. He was not responsive when asked to sit up, but he was still able to swallow, so I wriggled behind him to prop him up and let him sip orange juice. Within twenty minutes the orange juice worked its "magic" and we were able to communicate and he ate a full breakfast. It is amazing how the lack of such a small amount of glucose will cause the brain to malfunction to the point of semi-consciousness. Replace the missing glucose and within twenty minutes the brain is humming along.

Friday, January 23, 2004
 Midnight is truly the witching hour. Tonight the source of Jack's upset was the inability to get his partial denture out. He

kept pulling at his upper and lower teeth. He insisted it was in his mouth. but **they** did a lousy job and it was too tight.

Saturday, January 24- Tuesday, January 27, 2004

During the last few days, life has revolved around Jack's teeth. He keeps tugging at his teeth trying to get his partial out "because the left side of my face hurts." He has a sinus infection on that side and the pain is probably residual.

I don't think the partial is in his mouth but he won't let me look. However, I can't find it. I looked in the obvious places and most of the not-so-obvious places. Went piece by piece through every wastebasket and trash container.

Jack's talk turned to going to the dentist who would be able to get the partial out of his mouth. A heavy snow storm buried the area on Monday and into Tuesday. No one could travel, not us, not the dentist. It was a good thing because the dentist would have looked in his mouth and said, "What partial?"

Jack found it wrapped in tissue in a drawer. He had a hard time recognizing that it was his. He kept saying that it couldn't be his partial because you can't put teeth over teeth. Finally, I convinced him to try putting it into his mouth. It fit.

Tuesday, February 3, 2004

LaVerne had an appointment with her doctor today. She has been distraught over the recent death of a lifelong friend. Every phone conversation has been rambling and more repetitive than usual. Her perceptive doctor did cognitive testing and prescribed a medication for her for Alzheimer's Disease. It is not a cure. It slows the progression of symptoms.

LaVerne and her sister have the same doctor who then called and spoke to Lee at length about LaVerne's deteriorating mental condition. She said that she was not sure LaVerne was competent enough to drive. I have been wondering about this myself given the content of some of our phone conversations. Lee contends that LaVerne's driving skills are fine. Perhaps. But I know she is worried. If she admits that LaVerne cannot drive, she will become LaVerne's chauffeur.

Wednesday, February 4, 2004
Went down to the basement for sewing supplies and saw a little lake under the hot water heater. When the serviceman came to replace it, he asked where the main water shutoff valve was. Jack kept looking around and talking about something else. I pointed it out to the serviceman. Recently, I have noticed that when he is dealing with the public, Jack doesn't respond easily and appears unsure or confused. Sometimes, when he's asked a question, he starts talking about something that goes off on a related tangent but doesn't answer the question directly.

Tuesday, February 17, 2004
Tonight Jack was thoroughly confused about the date he wrote on a check. He has been saying, "When I worked, I always knew what day it was because I had a good calendar. I don't have anything now." All said while sitting at a drawing board that holds a clock with date and day of week, a 14x20-inch calendar pad with a page for each month and squares for each day, and a Disney calendar with a page for each day of the year.

Thursday, March 4, 2004
After dinner tonight, Jack asked why we missed going to Mass in the morning for his dad (date of death) and my mom (her birthdate). I explained that the date was next week. He looked at the calendar with uncertainty. "It was different when I

was working and had a calendar in front of me." He knew it was a Thursday, but not which one, not even when looking at the calendar.

Then he asked, "Tricia's birthday is on the 13th?" I was stunned by his question. Never did I think Jack would forget her birthday. The Irish daddy with the daughter born on St. Patrick's Day? Never!

I'm continuing to read everything I can find in print and on line about memory loss and its causes. Sometimes the cause is a simple imbalance in a substance necessary for brain functioning. I can vouch for that knowing how the lack of a little glucose can push a diabetic into a state of semi-consciousness. Replace the glucose and the person returns to full consciousness within twenty minutes.

There are also the more serious causes of memory loss: brain tumors, hydrocephalus, Parkinson's disease, as well as the dreaded Alzheimer's Disease. In Nathaniel Hawthorne's book, *The Scarlet Letter,* the "A" stood for adultery. Today, no one wants to be branded with the "A" that stands for Alzheimer's. A far more terrifying sentence.

March 5, 2004

At breakfast, Jack and I talked about the difficulties he was having in remembering and the possible causes. He agreed to see a specialist. An appointment has been made for March 19th.

Friday, March 19, 2004

At 7 a.m. this morning, Jack woke up and absolutely refused to go to the appointment scheduled for today. He was adamant. "There is nothing wrong with me. I am not crazy. Nobody is going to do anything with my head!" And that was that.

I am 99.9% sure he has Alzheimer's like his sister. But I wanted him to get the blood work done and an MRI to rule out other possibilities. If testing diagnosed a metabolic deficiency or other imbalance that could be corrected easily with supplements or medication, all his suffering would be over.

Sunday, March 28, 2004

Friends of ours were hosting a dinner at their home and invited us. One fellow was up here from Florida. His sister had just been diagnosed with Alzheimer's Disease. He was handling her affairs. Settling her into a secure residence where she would be safe and receive daily assistance with her needs. During the evening, I tried to question him discretely as to what behaviors or problems had confirmed the diagnosis. He had no definitive answers to give.

One of the other guests who is a nurse and long time friend of ours asked Jack how he was doing with his diabetes. She became thoroughly confused because he used the word *shot* interchangeably for blood glucose reading as well as insulin injection. She questioned him several times, then just gave up. Jack showed no sign of realizing that his responses did not make sense.

Monday, March 29, 2004

The amount of a check written out and a deposit were both added into the total in the checking account. When I mentioned this to Jack while balancing the checkbook, I sensed confusion about the error and an inability to understand why. Alzheimer's is muddying the waters of abstracts more and more, so amounts and dates are increasingly difficult.

Today, Jack made two bank deposits at different branches of the same bank. He is having difficulty in adding together all the checks to be deposited and then subtracting what he needs in cash for the month. He breaks it down because it is easier for him to handle. But he says that **they** would get it all mixed up if he deposited all of the checks at one time.

Jack is trying so hard to cope. He is smart enough to try getting around his difficulties by simplifying what he is doing. He pays bills immediately so due dates won't be bypassed and makes small deposits he can handle instead of one large one.

It tears at me to see him struggling. But any attempt to help irritates him. As long as things are not at the point of catastrophe, it's more important for him to feel he is still capable.

Tuesday, April 6, 2004

Jack received a letter stating that effective May 1st, his company insurance would no longer handle claims from the local hospital that we prefer to use. He was very upset, thinking he lost his insurance. A lot of explanation was needed to try and persuade him that it is only one hospital that is being dropped by the insurance company. It doesn't have any impact on doctor's office visits, prescription coverage, or patient services at other area hospitals.

He still called his endocrinologist's office and canceled his appointment for May 1st. Nothing that I said could convince him that Medicare and the insurance company would still pay their shares of the cost of the office visit, as they usually do.

At 4:30 p.m., a neighbor and I had a long standing date to see a movie and have dinner. It was a rare occasion and most enjoyable.

When I left the house, Jack had everything on the bed ready to change his glucometer to daylight savings time. I returned at 9:30 p.m. Everything had been moved to the kitchen table where the light is brighter. He was still trying to figure it out. It takes five minutes to reset the time. We did it together.

Wednesday, April 7, 2004

Called the endocrinologist's office to see if I could get an appointment for Jack before the end of April. Spoke to the nurse and explained the situation. She gave me an appointment for April 13th and said she would put a note in his file explaining the reason for the change. I am hoping his doctor will pick up on this and ask to speak to me. I'd still like to have testing done to rule out any other causes of memory loss.

Tuesday, April 13, 2004

Jack has started allowing me to accompany him to his appointments. I wait while he sees the doctor and then we go to a restaurant for lunch. Today, when he walked out of the exam room, he had trouble trying to repeat what the doctor told him.

Unfortunately, the doctor did not pick up on the content of the note and explore it further. It was a huge disappointment. If I made any attempt to talk to the doctor, Jack would be very irate. I need him to trust me completely and can't risk doing anything that would cause him to think I'm against him. It would make life unbearable for both of us.

Thursday, April 15, 2004

The battery for the new lawnmower was plugged in for recharging. When I asked Jack what time it should be unplugged, he said in all seriousness "when the hand is on the six." In the same vein, I asked him if it was the little hand or the big hand. He said, "You know, the hand." He could not tell the exact time.

Sunday, April 18, 2004

The credit card bill came with those pesky blank checks the company hopes one will use to pay off bills which are then added to the card. It caused concern that **they** were going to do something with the account. I offered to shred the checks but Jack was not convinced that the checks were harmless and decided to hang on to them for awhile because **they** are always up to something.

Saturday, May 1, 2004

Every so often, Jack enjoys playing the lottery and buys a ticket. Tonight he checked the numbers on his lottery ticket and said he didn't win even with the bonus numbers. When I asked what he meant by the bonus numbers, he pointed to the date of the lottery on the bottom of the ticket. It just makes me cry.

Sunday, May 2, 2004

Today the confusion was over the sentence on an invoice: "Enclose check or money order (no cash) payable to AARP." Three checks were written out putting that entire sentence on the Payable to line, instead of just the acronym AARP. There was frustration at not being able to write the check out properly. It was blamed on the way **they** made the invoice.

Monday, May 10, 2004

The mail brought the registration forms from the Village for cars and animals. Jack said, "Why do **they** send one for animals when we don't have any?" Lately, everything is becoming very personal to him. No amount of explanation can make him see that it is easier to include a form with all mailings since from year to year the Village really doesn't know who has pets, who doesn't, who has new pets, whose pets have died.

The registration forms have spawned a second concern. There are two forms, one for each car. Jack thinks he needs to make out two separate checks "because **they** are so screwed up, **they** won't know what to do if I give them one check." Again, he had difficulty writing the amounts in cursive. I do admire his determination to cope and save face. He can no longer figure out the total of the two forms, so he writes a separate check for each. If that helps him keep his dignity, why not! It also shows that other parts of the brain are still functioning quite well.

In the afternoon he made a deposit at the bank and asked for forty five-dollar bills because we are always in need of them. The difficulty was trying to figure out how much he had in total after they were put into eight piles of five bills per pile.

I know that Jack has Alzheimer's. Just wish it could be confirmed medically. But he is adamant about not going to see a neurologist. "I am not crazy. **They** are not going to do something with my head and mess it up." It is ironic. The mess is already there. *They* might be able to untangle it.

When Jack was growing up, there wasn't talk of dementias, autism, bipolar disorders, cognitive disabilities or mental health. A person who was slow or didn't act like everyone else was labeled: dumb, stupid, retarded, crazy, a dunce, an idiot. Few people wondered if there might be a medical problem affecting the brain that caused these behaviors.

Thursday May 13, 2004

Yesterday, Jack's ophthalmologist prescribed different eye drops to counteract the irritation he has been experiencing in his eyes. This morning he had the new bottle of eye drops sitting on the dresser in the bedroom. He said he was going to put them in his eyes. Reminded him they were only to be used once a day at bedtime. He disagreed and said he was supposed to use them twice a day. I showed him the information on dosage that had been written out for him on an index card as well as the dosage on the box from the eye drops.

We had a go-around. He kept saying he would go blind if he didn't put the drops in. I kept repeating that if he did that twice a day, he would damage his eyes. Finally, he put the drops away.

How I hate it when his doctors change something. It will be a good week before the new change is accepted. Until then, there will be frustration on both sides each day.

It is astounding to see how swiftly the frequency of these aberrations has accelerated. Everyday a new situation presents itself or an old one repeats itself. Each day is stress-filled. Even in the peaceful moments, I know that it is only a matter of time before another episode. When? Where? What? Why? I never know. What I do know without a doubt is that it will occur. So true relaxation is never possible. While Jack's brain is slowly disintegrating, mine is constantly calling on all its reserves to anticipate the next problem and prevent it, if possible.

"Cut 'em off at the pass" is my battle cry, just like in the old westerns.

Wednesday, May 19. 2004

While shopping today I mentioned that we needed a box of ice cream cones and started to look on the food shelves. Jack asked why I was looking there because they couldn't be on the shelf, they would melt. Explained that we needed plain ones to fill with ice cream at home. He still kept looking in the freezer.

At home, he said we should have gone to Baskin-Robbins and they would have fixed them. He couldn't picture cones without ice cream already in them. Yet, he is the one who fills all the ice cream cones at home!

Tuesday, May 25, 2004

Jack insisted on leaving home at 12:45 p.m. for a 2:30 p.m. appointment that Tricia had with the dentist. It only takes five to ten minutes to drive there. When she returned home, Tricia was not a happy camper since she had to wait almost two hours. She dislikes going to the dentist and the wait didn't help matters. At the dentist's, Jack used three checks before he got the amount right while trying to pay the bill. Tricia said his hand was shaking.

My poor Jack. What does he feel and understand about what is happening to him? How frightened he must be.

Wednesday, May 26, 2004

Today, while talking with LaVerne on the phone, she said, "Sometimes it feels like I am losing my mind."

There are increasing numbers of similarities between the actions of sister and brother. However, LaVerne's speech and communication skills are not impaired, whereas Jack's are. She can converse as always. And does. The only flaw is that each phone conversation is at least an hour long because she does not remember what she just said so each story is repeated over and over and over.

Jack does not repeat what he has said but he is rapidly losing the ability to process words. The avid fan of biographies and political tomes has not read a book in quite a while.

Saturday, June 5, 2004

Former President Ronald Reagan died this afternoon. He was ninety-three years old and had Alzheimer's Disease for at least twelve years. Ten years ago, he publicly announced that he had the disease. The immediate cause of death was pneumonia.

On the home front, Jack is happily spending all his time outside mowing the lawn and caring for the yard. The activity is good for him. He is busy with things he can still do without problems. And the sun and air tire him out in a good way.

Thursday, June 24, 2004

Jack and I started staining the siding on the house which is slurping up the gallons like a dehydrated puppy. He does the ladder work. He has never had a fear of heights, like I do. I'm a 6-runger at most, while he's scaled 40 footers with ease. Today, I noticed that his paintbrush was swinging erratically. Figured his blood glucose was low and mentioned it. Fortunately, he did not disagree with me. He managed to come down the ladder. But once on the ground, he started walking like a drunken sailor with me holding him up. Suddenly, he stopped in the middle of the wide open yard to move a stepladder so it won't be in the way. That made me laugh. Once inside the house, I did manage to get him into the kitchen and seated on a chair. A glass of orange juice and he was feeling much better in that magical twenty minutes.

People who have been diabetics for many years usually experience a lessening in their perception of when glucose is dropping in their system. The level can be quite low before the reaction is noticed by someone else. The loss of perception has nothing to do with memory loss. It is associated with the neuropathies that are complications of diabetes. However, the hypoglycemic reactions do complicate matters. Some of the first signs are irritation and fuzzy thinking, hallmarks of Alzheimer's. So the question then becomes, is this odd behavior the result of a hypoglycemic reaction or of a mental inability? Certainly does make life interesting!

Tuesday, July 20, 2004

Jack had his quarterly appointment with the endocrinologist. I purposely sat in the first chair in the waiting room hoping to get a chance to speak with his doctor without Jack's knowledge. He has adamantly refused to see any other doctor. I am desperate to get a medical opinion on the causes of his memory loss.

After his exam, I noticed that the doctor was leading Jack over to the area where blood is drawn. This was strange because the patients usually just walk there on their own. The nurse had another patient so she asked Jack to sit in the waiting room until he was called. He came and sat down next to me and told me he had a reading of 126. I wondered how he could know what it was before the blood work was done. He said the doctor wanted him to bring his meter in for a recheck because Jack had told him about all the low readings. Jack said he told the doctor he had to have lunch and the doctor told him that was okay. He could bring it in the afternoon.

As we were talking, I noticed the endocrinologist coming out toward Jack. He noticed us talking, paused a moment and then seemed relieved as he walked toward us. Since we had never met, I put out my hand and introduced myself. When he found out that I was Jack's wife, he started to say something, stopped, and then asked if he could have a word with me. We went into the examining room.

He started by saying that he was totally confused by what Jack was trying to tell him, that Jack had been like this before (April visit), that he hadn't followed through on what the doctor had asked him to do, and that what Jack was saying didn't make sense. He said he took a glucose reading and it was 126 - normal range. (So that explained what Jack said.) He initially thought the incoherence might be the result of a hypoglycemic reaction.

I replied that through all our married years, anytime I noticed speech or actions that were a bit odd or abnormal, I automatically assumed that Jack was having a reaction. And testing would prove it.

Now I could no longer make that assumption. Often the oddities have no relation to the glucose level. And it is harder because I can't just ask Jack to take a reading, so I know for sure. If he is upset already, asking him to do that just adds fuel to the fire. So I have to observe more closely and guess.

We spoke for more than twenty minutes. For me, it was like opening the flood gates. Finally I had someone to whom I could mention the changes and losses and my concerns and suspicions and fears. He suggested that Jack see a neurologist for cognitive testing. I informed him of the aborted appointment at the mental health center.

When we returned with the glucometer, the endocrinologist told Jack to test his glucose four times a day and to take ten units of insulin in the morning and at dinnertime. No more than that. Jack said, "But what if I am low?" The doctor replied, "Then you will need to drink some orange juice. If you are low, you do not need insulin."

On the way home, Jack kept saying, "The guy is going to kill me and you have to watch out. He wants me to take ten units of insulin four times a day." And I kept replying, " He wants you to take a reading four times a day and only ten units of insulin – no more - two times a day."

Wednesday, July 21, 2004

At lunch today, Jack pulled the insulin out of the fridge. He said that he was supposed to take ten units. Reminded him that the endocrinologist wanted him to take a reading four times a day. Insulin was only taken twice like he had always been doing. Again, we went over and over the instructions. This is going to be a l-o-n-g week.

Monday, July 26, 2004

One of my brothers-in-law had a fatal heart attack early this morning. It was a blessing. His lung cancer had returned and he had several inoperable clogged arteries. My oldest sister was not prepared for this. The day was spent on the phone with her as well as calling all the other members of the family.

Thursday, July 29, 2004

After the Mass and the service at the cemetery, we visited the graves of my mom and dad, grandparents, uncles, aunts. It has been several years since I was there. No one lives in the area anymore and it is a drive of over sixty miles.

Except for my brother Frank, I have not seen any other members of my family since my birthday party last September. Mixed in with the sadness of the occasion was the joy of seeing everyone and noticing the growth spurts of my grandnieces and grandnephews. It was good to chat face to face with my sisters over lunch and catch up on the tidbits that never seem to make it into our often suddenly abbreviated phone conversations.

Jack listened more than spoke. I noticed that sometimes he could not follow the conversations. Overall, he was having a good day for which I am most grateful. Thank you, dear Lord, for allowing me to be part of this family memory.

The drive home was quite stressfilled because there was construction on the road and the usual afternoon traffic. Jack asked me if there was anyone else in the family who would be buried at that far away cemetery. When I started to name several relatives, he just shook his head.

Sunday, August 8, 2004

Today was the annual family reunion at my cousin Tom's home, another fifty-mile drive. Jack was quiet while we were there. None of the usual going-off-in-a-corner with one of the guys and conversing for hours or making small talk with a group at table. He just sat in a chair with one hand on top of the other.

The drive home was hairy and scary. We had hoped to leave at 7 p.m. so the drive would be in daylight. It was almost 8 p.m. when we left and the sun was setting. There were dark areas on some of the roads which made it difficult to see clearly. On the expressway, I could see by the set of his jaw that the driving was not easy for Jack. Fortunately, there was little traffic. He drove with good skill. Only when we came into the subdivision, did he start to go over a curb and almost hit a small tree.

Once home, I noticed that his forehead was hot and took his temperature. It was 102°. That explained the difficulty in driving tonight. However, it is time to stay close to home. His driving skills are still excellent. But the long distances are too stressful. I could see that two weeks ago when we went to the funeral. A long drive requires a long period of concentration. And that is no longer easily done.

Tuesday, August 10, 2004

Jack did not know that today was my birthday. Usually a week or two before, he will ask where I want to go for dinner. This year he did not.

All day the phone kept ringing with people wishing me a happy day. He didn't seem to realize what was occurring and never asked why the phone kept ringing and who was calling. Even Tricia couldn't figure it out. She wanted to know what we were going to do for dinner. I told her that if Daddy didn't offer to dine out because he didn't remember it was my birthday, I would order dinner and have it delivered.

Around 4 p.m., the phone rang yet again and Jack asked me why the phone kept ringing. I explained that people were calling to wish me a happy birthday.

He looked puzzled, "But I thought your birthday was the first, in the future."

"The first of October?"

"Yes."

"Honey, that's our anniversary."

I mentioned ordering dinner for delivery. He immediately insisted that we order ribs and shrimp and all my favorite dishes and especially a cake for dessert.

When Jack did not mention my birthday during this past week, I decided to say nothing and use it as a test to see if he had truly forgotten. But after seeing the look on his face when he realized that he had forgotten it, I will never do that again. I will drop gentle hints so that his self-esteem isn't hurt by what his erratic brain is doing.

Thursday, August 12, 2004

LaVerne called all eager to tell me something she had told me several times in the past week. After I hung up, Jack asked what the call was all about. He said, "I wonder if she has that disease that seems to be affecting everyone - you know, like that actor...you know, the one with the guns and the president who died, you know...that disease they keep talking about so much, that Al, Alz..."

I said, "You mean Alzheimer's?"

He said, "Yes."

I told him she did. I wonder if he worries internally about whether it is his problem. One just doesn't know what is going on in the mind of a person afflicted with it.

For the first time in our marriage, there is a topic we cannot discuss. The slightest mention of anything not being right just triggers agitation. It is not worth it. As long as I am reasonably sure what is happening and what I can do to make life easier for him, I'm content. Jack does not need to know. It would only hurt him.

Friday, August 13, 2004

Something new. This morning Jack asked me to tally up the bank deposit "so I don't get it wrong." A year ago, he never would have asked me to do that, nor would he have needed to ask.

Sunday, August 15, 2004

We are now attending the early Mass on Sunday morning rather than the one on Saturday afternoon. It is quieter and easier for Jack.

After Mass, we drove out to LaVerne's so I could go over paperwork with her. She is an absolute basket case because her TV is not working. She does realize her mind is failing her and she is terrified of the future. I suggested that a private apartment in a building for seniors might be a good idea. She said she would be fearful of meeting the other people and she meant it. The look on her face was sheer terror.

Monday, August 30, 2004

In a phone conversation with LaVerne, she mentioned how she had always sent contributions to the Alzheimer's Association because she thought it was such a terrible disease. She said she didn't know much about it other than what she read or heard and now she has it. This is the first time that she has verbally made that acknowledgment.

Wednesday, September 7, 2004

On Friday, the notice came for the emissions testing on the 1998 Mercury. Jack was obsessed with the notice all Labor Day weekend. He was positive that the car wouldn't pass. We had the car tested this morning. The test was a breeze and we were done in five minutes. A-OK.

The purchase of the car was the first odd occurrence involving Jack that puzzled me. In thirty years of marriage, we had only purchased four cars. Each time Jack decided what make and model he wanted. Then, over a period of one or two weeks, we visited every showroom that had that make and model, some more than once. He went over every inch of every vehicle in which he was interested. It tried my patience as well as that of every hopeful salesman. Finally, he would make a decision.

In August 1998, as dealerships were moving out the '98's at great prices to make room for the new '99's, Jack decided it was time to trade in the mileage laden station wagon that we had used to haul the inventory for the doll shows. He announced that he wanted a silver 1998 Mercury Marquis.

The very next morning, he was up early and dressed and ready to go to the dealership he selected as soon as it opened. As we walked into the showroom, there was his car lording it over all the other cars on the showroom floor. Jack sat inside, looked it over and began talking with the salesman who was mentally calculating his fat commission. As they spoke, I slid into the driver's seat and looked around. This supposedly brand new showroom floor car had two hundred fifty-seven miles on the odometer. Hmmm.

After the salesman walked to the office to get the contract, I mentioned the mileage to Jack. This car had been driven. When the salesman rejoined us, Jack asked him to pop the hood, something he had not thought to have him do earlier. Everything under the hood looked like it had been in a dust storm. This car had been driven to Illinois from a dealership in a neighboring state. That was a deal breaker for Jack.

As we drove toward home, he mentioned another Mercury dealership. He was intent on driving directly there. It was almost noon. He needed a meal. Let's go after lunch.

While we ate, the sunny morning disappeared, pushed out of the way by menacing gray clouds. The visit to the dealership would have to wait until tomorrow. Surprisingly, as soon as Jack finished his ham sandwich, he was ready to go. The storm was imminent but it didn't faze him. Definitely, not like Jack.

As we drove to the dealership the sky took on a tinge of green, thunder began rolling and lightning flashed. We had just parked at the dealership and ran inside when the rain began to pour down. For twenty minutes we sat next to a salesman's desk while sheets of rain obliterated everything outside the windows, the lights flickered and lightning strikes close by shook the building. Whatever were we doing?

The storm rolled east, and the western sky began to clear. A mechanic went out to the lot to bring in a silver Marquis. It was dried off so we could inspect it. The odometer registered six miles and the engine gleamed. For Jack it was a done deal. Happily, he drove out of the dealership in the brand new car he had bought in one day. A first for him. A puzzlement for me.

Sunday, September 19, 2004

LaVerne called. She was very upset. As near as I could figure out from her incoherent rambling, she had lost her car keys while attending a picnic at her sister's condo complex. They searched everywhere and could not find them. She had to stay overnight because her car was parked in front of the garage and Lee couldn't get out. In the morning a friend drove them to LaVerne's, so she could get the second set of keys and move her car.

Tuesday, September 21, 2004

Spent over two hours on the phone tonight with LaVerne. She remembers none of what happened two days ago. She said she had trouble with the key fitting the lock in her car and she had spent the day looking for her second set of keys. I tried explaining over and over that that was the second set of keys that she had. She had lost the first set. She needed to have another set of keys made just in case this set was lost or misplaced. She must do it tomorrow.

After two hours of repetition, she still was confused. My only hope is that she will have duplicates of the keys made. If it happened once, it will happen again. Without backup keys, the situation will be even more stressful.

Thursday, September 23, 2004

The endocrinologist wanted to know why Jack hadn't seen the neurologist. I reminded him that my attempt last year had failed and that I had asked him to talk to Jack about it. He went over to the blood testing station and talked to Jack, who told him in no uncertain terms that he wasn't crazy, he was getting along well and if the doctor wanted to give me the name, fine, but he wasn't going.

He isn't crazy. The dementia is something over which he has no control. It would be interesting to have a battery of tests which might pinpoint the areas of strength as well as areas of weakness. It would be an immense help in everyday life.

On the other hand, if the subject of the tests isn't fully cooperative, the results would be skewed and worth very little. What good will it do to go through hell just to confirm what I already know.

Saturday, September 25, 2004

What a stressful day! Drove out to LaVerne's and had new sets of car keys made for her car at the hardware store in town. We went to lunch at a little café. She couldn't make up her mind what she wanted. Really don't think she understands the menu anymore. She enjoys BLT's so I decided to order that and suggested that she do the same. She enjoyed every bite. The medication for Alzheimer's has depressed her appetite and she eats very little. However, with some coaxing she did quite well.

In the process of looking over the annuity that she was talked into at a bank, I found that she had filed last month's credit card bill without paying it. Wrote out a check for the bill and she signed it. Took the annuity paperwork home with me. Will call during the week to see what can be done to void it. Any one who talks to her for more than a few minutes can see that her grasp of numbers is tenuous. It angers me that someone would take advantage of her and allow her to sign these annuity papers.

Tuesday, September 28, 2004
Situations that include numbers are also a stumbling block for Jack - setting the alarm, dealing with bills, dating the sheets for blood glucose readings. Jack said that "it didn't seem right that 9/28 comes after 9/27. It is all screwed up."

It took him over two hours to write two checks. On one envelope, he wrote his name and address, then stopped and said, "**They** are so sloppy and didn't put the zip code on there." Reminded him that it was his address and his zip code, not the company's.

Friday, October 1, 2004
Today is our 38th wedding anniversary. This morning Jack went out early and came home with three huge bouquets of flowers.

Tricia was puzzled when her dad gave her a box of candy - and a Sweetest Day card. Then Jack gave me a box of candy and the most beautifully composed card with a message I will treasure always - wishing me a Happy Birthday. My heart bled. But he looked so pleased with himself and was happy. What did it matter?

Last week when we were talking about going out for dinner, he asked, "It isn't your birthday, is it?"

I replied, "No, that was in August."

He said, "I didn't think so."

But gave no clue that he knew it was our anniversary.

Tuesday, October 5, 2004

The Grand Victoria casino boat is celebrating its Tenth Anniversary and sent Jack an invitation which includes a free buffet lunch. He wanted to go and see what the machines were like now that they gave tickets to winners instead of coins. We looked at the machines together and I showed him how they worked. It was easy and he caught on without too much trouble. We stayed together and had fun.

The buffet lunch had choices of salad, Italian, Oriental, and Mexican food as well as all the traditional American meats and vegetables, and an outstanding array of fruits, ice creams and desserts. We found a table by the windows with the sun warm upon us and enjoyed a leisurely lunch.

After lunch, we returned to the casino. Jack took off so fast, I lost track of him in the throng of people. It took a while to maneuver through everyone and check both floors. When I finally found him, he was playing a Slots for Dummies machine. I stayed with him watching him play and having fun. The machine really paid off on several jackpots and he won $475. Earlier I had won $250. We left the casino with over $700.

Winning was good, but what was even better was that we both had a day together that was so calm and easy. It has been a long time since the last one. I am grateful.

Friday, October 15, 2004

The lottery is the latest nemesis. Jack filled out two forms and seemed to understand how many numbers he needed to pick for each one. Still he came home upset because **they** couldn't give him the tickets. He had picked the correct numbers on each form, but also marked off the box for quick picks. Either you pick your own numbers or have the machine do it for you as a quick pick. Marking both voids the form because the machine can't do both. There was nothing the cashier could do about it.

Friday, October 29, 2004

I am reading a book about two professors and the wife's Alzheimer's. Just finished a section on how the good days or moments had the husband doubting the diagnosis and feeling everything is fine, until something happened again and he knew his wife was not okay. How I can empathize with him.

Just as I closed the book, Jack came into the workroom with a slip of paper on which he had written in cursive the amount of the gas bill. It was correct. However, he wrote the check out wrong and had to start over, a common occurrence these days. Our once pristine checkbook, the work of his hands and of which he had been so proud, has turned into a hodgepodge of voided checks and rewritten numbers. Sigh.

Monday, November 1, 2004

Up at 7 a.m. on a rainy day. After breakfast, I noticed that Jack was all dressed up with his coat and hat on the bed. I asked him where he was going.

He said, "Aren't you going anywhere?"

"No. Where are you going?"

"To vote."

"Tomorrow is election day."

"**They** are always screwing everything up. The people in Florida can vote early."

The concept of time has disappeared. All week long he kept questioning when Tricia and I have our dental appointments and when he has his appointment with the endocrinologist, which is not until December 20th.

Friday, November 12, 2004

Yesterday afternoon, Jack cut the grass for the last time this year. Then he went into the bedroom and shut the door. He does this when he wants privacy using the phone. Three hours went by. I assumed he fell asleep on the bed.

I knocked on the door, then walked into the bedroom to get a heavy jacket before taking a walk. He was sitting in the rocker going over a women's specialty catalog. He had spent three hours trying to figure out what he needed to do to place an order.

When I returned from the walk, we spent the evening going over the steps for placing an order. And all of this morning.

This afternoon he called and placed his order. Afterward he said he wasn't sure what he ordered. What a difference this year has made. Last year he outdid himself ordering from catalogs.

Friday, November 19, 2004

Today, Tricia and I were talking with her dad about going out to dinner on Sunday for his birthday and having dinner at home on Monday, which is the actual birthdate. She has to work on Monday. While talking about Sunday, he said, "But isn't that Easter?" Even after saying it, he didn't recognize the mistake.

He is still aware that a holiday is close at hand, but he is no longer sure of which one or when. His birthday is the twenty-second of November, celebrated very close to Thanksgiving and every so many years on the holiday itself.

Sunday, November 21, 2004

Since August we have been going to the 7:30 a.m. Mass on Sunday mornings. This has worked well, except for one thing. Jack gets up at 3 or 4 a.m. in the morning to get ready. His sense of time is so elusive and he worries about being late.

Early in the afternoon we went for a most enjoyable dinner. The food was excellent and the atmosphere was relaxed. As we were leaving the restaurant, Jack asked, "Is today my birthday or tomorrow?" That shattered my heart into a thousand pieces.

Monday, November 22, 2004

Jack's seventy-fifth birthday. Since Tricia was working, we gave him his birthday gifts at lunch time. He was pleased with the gifts but not sure why he was receiving them. Even wishing him a Happy Birthday was met with uncertainty. At dinnertime, when he came into the kitchen and asked what I was fixing and heard lobster, his face lit up like that of an innocent young boy. He ate his dinner with the same gusto.

Monday, November 29, 2004

Today the three of us made our traditional Monday after Thanksgiving trip to Woodfield Mall to do Christmas shopping. We arrive early in the morning and put our coats in a locker. We split up until 11 o'clock when we meet in the mall's center court on the upper level. We have lunch, then split up again until about 4 o'clock. We meet again in the center court, collect our coats and head for home.

Tricia and I were at the checkout in Sears when we saw Jack hurrying toward us as fast as he could. He was frantic. He said he'd been in every store two or three times looking for us because he didn't know where we were supposed to meet. He thought he'd have to call the police. I walked with him to our meeting place where we could sit down and encouraged Tricia to do whatever shopping she could and meet us there. Jack sat on the bench totally drained of energy.

Another heartbreaker. He selected that meeting place over a dozen years ago and we've used it ever since.

Wednesday, December 1, 2004

Today is twenty-five years since Jack's mom died. The three of us attended a Mass celebrated in her memory, then went to breakfast afterward.

Later in the day, my brother Frank called to invite us to the family holiday gathering on January 1st. Since all the members of my family live at least fifty miles away, we do not see each other often. It was difficult to refuse an invitation. Earlier in the year, we did not go to two parties celebrating First Communions because Jack was not up to it.

Because my family only sees us two or three times a year, they have not noticed the significant changes in Jack. I have begun to tell them that he has Alzheimer's. Since they have not seen the decline, some are skeptical and think I am overreacting. Their thinking is actually not much different than mine was when I noticed the first little changes.

Frank and I may not see each other often, but we are close in mind and heart. We connect by phone at least once a week, usually when he is snailing his way home on the expressways. He has been aware of my concerns for some time. He was not surprised when I told him I did not think we could make the trip. I asked him to please make other family members aware that this is serious, and our not attending is more than a whim.

He suggested coming up to visit on the day after Christmas, an idea I eagerly embraced. In one respect, it has always been lonely being so far from family. But that was tempered by the close relationship Jack and I have had. We were content with each other. Now I am losing him bit by bit. It is just lonely.

Wednesday, December 15, 2004
Busy time of year. Jack pulled the tree and the holiday decorations out of the crawl space and the house looks lovely draped in green and red and gold.

Tricia and I went to the local high school craft fair on Saturday. It was so different to be on the customer side of the booth. It was enjoyable having a chance to chat with other crafters. Usually, when I did the shows, I didn't have time.

Frank confirmed that he will be coming out on the 26th with his family. I am happy.

Monday, December 20, 2004

With his permission, I can now accompany Jack into the examining room for his medical appointments. I translate what Jack is saying for the doctor and know what the doctor is doing.

It has had another advantage. I noticed that the doctor used a modern glucometer. Instead of putting in a strip one at a time, a drum of strips is inserted and the meter will automatically pull one out of the drum for each blood glucose reading. Also, the meter does not have to be coded for each new batch of strips. Jack is having so much trouble with this but still insists that he has always done it on his own and can still do it.

I asked the doctor if Jack could use a meter like that at home. He agreed and gave one to me that was a free sample from the pharmaceutical company. I know that Jack will resist using it and probably will not remember how to use it on his own. But it might be the answer to being allowed to help him with his readings and injections. Being there, I will know for sure how much insulin he is taking. Right now, I still have to guess. Jack writes the numbers down on the chart, but it is becoming more and more jumbled and difficult to figure out. This may be the solution.

Friday, December 24, 2004

This is the first Christmas Eve in twenty-five years that we have not attended the Christmas Eve Mass. Since we need to go to church in the morning and LaVerne is coming for Christmas Day dinner, I told Tricia that we would open our gifts tonight. She is a traditionalist and reminded me that we always open them on Christmas morning. She doesn't like to change things but accepts it because she knows that the changes are made so it will be easier for her dad.

And things do change. With his artist's eye and penchant for perfection, in years past, all of Jack's gifts were wrapped so perfectly that one didn't want to open them and spoil the beauty. He always teased me about the many ways he could wrap ribbon around a package that I could not.

Last year, Jack was wrapping his gifts when I left to go shopping one morning. When I returned at dinnertime, he was still busy wrapping. Tricia said he had been at it all day. He was exhausted and said he still had a lot to do. Never had it taken him so long. On Christmas morn, the gifts were beautifully wrapped and I really did hate to open them knowing how much effort had been expended.

This year, his ability was diminished. The effort was made to still wrap everything but the techniques were missing. It made no difference. Tonight after dinner, we settled in the living room by the tree and exchanged gifts. It was very cozy and relaxing. At last, I was able to see the items that Jack had so much trouble ordering in November. He did well.

As we were cleaning up paper and bows, Tricia asked me why her dad signed her card so funny. She gave me the card. Instead of signing it as he always did "Love, Daddy", he had signed it "Your Father, Jack."

Saturday, December 25, 2004

A most interesting Christmas. The three of us attended Christmas Mass at 9 a.m. It was a different experience seeing the celebration in the light of day. The Mass was not overcrowded, so it was good for Jack.

Just before we left for church, LaVerne called. She wanted to know why a friend of hers had called and told her she needed to get up and go to church. I told her it was Christmas morning.

"But why do I have to go?" Round and round we went. I was ready to tell her to forget it, when she said that she would get dressed and go. I told her to call me when she returned home. I did not want to confuse her by giving her any more information.

Every year LaVerne has driven out on Christmas Day to have dinner with us, while her sister is visiting her daughter on the east coast. She comes in the early afternoon and stays until nine or ten o'clock. This year I did not want her driving. It is a distance of thirty miles and I am not sure she remembers the way. She is becoming more and more confused. It frightens me to think of her being alone in the car on a cold, snowy night and not knowing where she is.

LaVerne did call back. I told her that I had ordered a cab to pick her up and bring her here for Christmas dinner. She should bring her nightgown and makeup and medicine because she would stay overnight. Frank would take her home tomorrow. She said taking a cab would be too much money. She would give the driver directions so it wouldn't cost so much. I told her to just sit back in the cab and let the cabbie do the driving.

About 3 p.m., the phone rang as I was preparing dinner. It was a harried cab driver. He said he had a very agitated lady in the back seat. Could I tell him how to get to our house? He was at the Deerfield Toll Plaza. I gave him instructions on how to get here from there.

He told me he was originally going to take the Tristate expressway to I-290 to Route 53. He said the lady kept telling him it was the wrong way. She'd been here a thousand times and knew how to come. When he realized he was in Lake County, he knew he had gone too far.

In a few minutes the phone rang again. It was the cabbie. He was on Lake-Cook Road and wasn't sure how to proceed from there. Once he had the directions, he asked if I would please come out when he arrived. Assured him I had intended to do that.

When he pulled into the driveway, the cabbie rolled his eyes and shook his head. He whispered, "I have never had a passenger like this." Meanwhile, LaVerne gathered her belongings and got out of the cab. All the while she was motioning and mumbling that the guy did not know what he was doing. What should have been a $60 cab fare was $100+ with the side trip to Deerfield!

Once LaVerne calmed down and forgot about the incident, the day was fine. Since the conversation never focused on the past, she and Jack had no need to get testy with each other.

In our home there was Christmas peace on earth, a treasure to be cherished.

Sunday, December 26, 2004

An extension of Christmas day with Frank's family joining us for dinner. It was good to have time to visit with them alone. We usually only see each other at large family gatherings where one-on-one conversations never seem to work.

LaVerne was so delighted to have Frank drive her home. Immediately, she called me to say how smart he was. He knew exactly how to get to her house. She never realized how good-looking he was. If she were younger, she'd be interested. Some things never change!

Monday, December 27, 2004

I decided to call the cab company and commend the driver who brought LaVerne here on Christmas Day. When I reached the dispatcher and told him my purpose, he was delighted that someone would call to give recognition and said that he would put it out on the airwaves immediately.

Cabbies were used to dealing with all kinds of people, but someone with Alzheimer's might be unusual. He said that the company has had other passengers with similar problems. He related that on Thanksgiving, a cabbie picked up a woman who was going to her son's home for dinner. Three hours later she had not shown up and the family was frantic. The cab company had to put out an all-points bulletin to be on the lookout for the cab. When the cab was finally spotted, the driver said the woman was very agitated and threatened him with her cane. She, too, kept telling him what streets to use and where to turn until both were totally lost.

Friday, December 31, 2004

This has been a year of significant losses for Jack. What I questioned one year ago, today is fact. There is no doubt in my mind that Alzheimer's is claiming Jack as one of its victims. The pace has accelerated. Every day now there is some oddity or confusion or slippage. The scary part is that I am growing so accustomed to this that it almost seems normal in the pattern of day-to-day living. I must not let that happen.

◊◊◊◊◊◊◊◊◊◊

CHAPTER SEVEN

Saturday, January 1, 2005

A quiet beginning to another new year. Just the three of us together. While the surface may look quiet, fear and anxiety are bubbling furiously underneath. So much changed last year. What will happen this year?

Thursday, January 6, 2005

It started snowing heavily yesterday and continued on through this morning. Jack has used the snow blower several times. Now he and Tricia are outside shoveling snow off the evergreens and the roof. It is good exercise for him, which should help his circulation and mental functioning. I do worry a bit about the possibility of a fatal heart attack. But would that be worse than what is claiming him now?

Monday, January 17, 2005

I knew the calmness of the past ten days couldn't last. Jack is still taking the checks to the bank one at a time. He has given me various reasons why. "That Mickey Mouse bank can't handle it." "**They** will mess it up." In the process of doing this, he gets so confused trying to figure out how much cash he wants to take out of each check. But he insists on doing it.

Throughout these past five years, Jack has been fighting a quixotic battle with **"they"**. In this case, **they** are the doctors and pharmacists and banks and companies, etc. With a mind unable to deal with a situation or problem - any situation or problem - **they** have become the scapegoat.. **They** are the source of all this aggravation and frustration. If **they** did their jobs properly, his life would be wonderful. While it is frustrating to be the recipient of long harangues about **they** each time something isn't right, there is a silver lining. **"They"** could have been "you" - meaning me!

Monday, January 24, 2005

For the past few days the '85 Chevy won't start. The lights function, it makes a noise, but the engine will not turnover.

Jack was going to try taking the battery out and getting a replacement but he is concerned that the hookup will not be the same. That concern is a good sign that parts of his brain are still functioning well. I am relieved that he isn't insisting on doing it himself.

He has always been "Jack" of all trades, trying to save money. For many years he had to because finances were tight. But often he'd get into a situation that would take him forever and cause a lot of tension because he didn't have the proper tools or equipment or hardware, etc. Eventually he always resolved the problem. But something a professional would have done in twenty minutes would take him all day, sweating and straining and running back and forth to the hardware stores.

This morning he called the local service station and was embarrassed because he could not remember his home phone number when asked.

When the fellow came from the service station with the tow truck, I noticed how slow Jack was in understanding what the young guy was telling him. It is so sad to see how much he has declined in a year.

The fellow did well because the car was in the garage very close to the door frame and he had to get it out and tow it. He put it in neutral and asked Jack to steer it while he pushed it out with ease.

Then he told Jack to put it into park which he did. The guy was going to bring the tow truck into the driveway. But Jack put the car back in neutral and it slid down too far for the tow truck to get behind it. The fellow had to push the car out into the street and turn it to face south. Jack tried to help push but he has no strength and the car got stuck at the bottom of the driveway.

Another young guy in an SUV was coming down the street. He took in the situation, stopped, and asked the tow truck driver if he needed help. The two young guys easily got the car into position. The tow truck driver patted his helper on the back and said, "Thanks, man." The guy got back in his SUV and took off. From there it was easy to get the car onto the tow truck.

When we came into the house, Jack said the tow truck driver wasn't too smart. He wouldn't listen to what Jack thought he should do. He doesn't realize that he is doing exactly what LaVerne would do, which irritated him. For years she would ask Jack to fix something in her house. Then she wouldn't let him alone and kept telling him how to do it. That's probably what the tow truck driver thought.

As I watched, I couldn't help thinking,"Young man, how I wish you could see my man when he was your age. He was like you. Now you only see the slowness and the age and ignore him. But pay attention, because once he was young and strong like you. Someday, only too soon, you will be like him."

Saturday, February 12, 2005

Jack and I drove out to LaVerne's to get her income tax papers together. All her adult life, she has been very savvy with her finances, buying and selling stocks and bonds, not only for the firm where she worked but also for herself.

Now she is rapidly losing her grip on what is what. It would have been impossible for her to do this on her own, another decline since a year ago. She said it was hard to do it last year, but she did it. By summertime she said paperwork was no longer the joy it had once been. By fall, she needed help. Now just asking for a certain Form 1099 is greeted with uncertainty.

Last night she mentioned to me that the light on the pole outside the garage was burnt out. She was afraid to get on a ladder to replace it. She no longer takes chances since she fell off the stepstool and broke her wrist. No more high wire acts climbing up on the roof to clean gutters.

We took bulbs with us because she never has any and we weren't sure of the wattage. Jack tried several bulbs but couldn't get the light to work. He said he didn't know what else to do. In passing, I asked if he checked the fuse box, then went back to my task. I knew the taxes would take a long time and we needed to leave while it was still light outside.

After I finished getting the tax info in order, I heard Jack and LaVerne talking about the light and getting an electrician. I decided to go down to the basement and check the fuse box. The lights for the laundry room wouldn't work. When I located the fuse box using a flashlight, I noticed one breaker was tripped. I flipped it on and the basement lights went on. The sump pump kicked in. Within a minute, the breaker tripped off. Each time I tried it, the same thing happened. An electrician was a must.

LaVerne was beside herself. I was wishing I had checked it earlier so an electrician would have come while I was there. It was also 3 p.m. on a Saturday. With the grace of God, I looked through the yellow pages and found an electrician who would be out within a half hour.

It is heartbreaking to see how much Jack is slipping. In the past, no problem ever eluded him. A year ago, he would have checked the fuse box first thing when the bulbs didn't work. Now it never occurred to him. He just sat in a chair with his hands folded waiting patiently while I did the paperwork.

I told LaVerne I would call as soon as we arrived home. I did. The electrician was there and she gave the phone to him. He explained that the sump pump was drawing 23 amps on a 15 amp fuse. A new pump was needed. Approved replacing the pump and asked him to check the outdoor light which started the whole thing. By 8 p.m., LaVerne was back in business with a new sump pump and a bright light.

Sunday, February 13, 2005

At lunch today, Jack kept asking if tomorrow was Tricia's birthday. Reminded him her birthday is March 17, St. Patrick's Day. Tomorrow is Valentines Day.

Monday, February 14, 2005

Jack went out in the morning. He had filled out a lottery ticket, but once again, it was wrong. He was aggravated because "**they** never get it right."

He gave me a card that said Thinking of You. And once again he signed a card for Tricia "From your Father, Jack", instead of "Love, Daddy."

He is losing so much, it is both sad and scary. But he still remembered the cards, a definite plus.

February 26, 2005

More lotto mayhem. Jack finally filled out a form for the lottery with his own numbers and got it right.

After the drawing tonight, he came into the family room all excited and smiling. "I won $20 million!! Look at this, I have all the numbers." He was comparing the lotto form he filled out and the printed ticket he bought at the store. "Every number is there! I won 20 million dollars!!"

He didn't understand that he needed to check the printed ticket against the numbers picked on TV. He was going to the store in the morning with his winning ticket. He was positive he had won. All night he tossed and turned and hardly slept a wink. Neither one of us did. Jack because he was so excited and me because I was dreading the humiliation he would experience in the morning when he took the ticket to the store insisting that he had won $20 million.

First thing before breakfast, I checked the ticket against the numbers in the newspaper. Jack's ticket had three numbers in one row, so there was a small win. After breakfast, I went to the store with him. He was so insistent that he won, I wasn't sure how he would react with the clerk.

I could tell that what he was saying made no sense to her. But she did say that no one had won the big prize. Finally, she scanned the ticket and gave him $3.

My silent prayers were answered when he accepted the small amount quietly. I could see by the way he shook his head that he couldn't quite understand why. Another heartbreaker.

Wednesday, March 9, 2005

This evening there was confusion between the vial of insulin and bottle of eye drops. Both are in identical sized boxes in the fridge. Jack pulled out the box with the eye drops bottle at dinnertime instead of the insulin. He panicked and said, "**They** gave me the wrong thing." He thought he didn't have insulin and what would he do. I can't always figure out how his mind is processing things. He failed to identify the different information on each box and the differences in the bottles.

Monday, March 14, 2005

Last fall Jack's credit card company made an agreement with another company and offered an exclusive credit card to select customers. Jack was one of them. When the new card came, he was aggravated. He called the company. The service rep told him it was a better card. He could use it just like the old one.

The cover letter that accompanied the new credit card indicated that if a person spent a thousand dollars on the new card by December 31, 2014, a fifty-dollar gift card would be sent as a Thank You for using the new card. A marketing ploy. The card was used for groceries and gifts all fall and through the holidays, so the thousand dollars was easily reached.

Today the gift card came and there was instant aggravation. Jack thought it was another new card and **they** said that if you spend more than fifty dollars, you can't use it and **they** want you to travel. What the letter did say was that anything over and above fifty dollars would be charged to your credit card and you couldn't use it for airlines, hotels or gas.

I tried explaining that if he didn't use it, it would be like throwing a fifty-dollar bill in the trash. It was a gift. He said that if that's what I thought, I was a sucker. **They** want you to think that but he's smarter than that. He's going to call in the morning and tell **them** he doesn't want the new card. Could not convince him otherwise.

Tuesday, March 15, 2005

Not a good day. At breakfast Jack said he didn't sleep at all last night because of the card. Shortly thereafter, he decided to call the credit card company. I had to redial the number because the first thing they asked for was his credit card number and he did not understand that meant the other one in his wallet, not the gift card.

Would have loved to hear that whole conversation with the customer service rep wanting to know *why* he didn't want a gift card.

The issue was resolved when the rep said she would cancel the new credit card and send another like his old one. The gift card was still his to use.

Thursday, March 17, 2005
St. Patrick's Day and Tricia's birthday. It was a quiet one. She will celebrate with her friends on the weekend.
Her dad and I treated her at the local restaurant staffed by singing waiters. The food is excellent. My two Irishmen by birth won't touch corned beef and cabbage, so I never fix it. I savored a plate of the same while they ordered steak and chicken with salad. The Irish singers saluted Tricia's birthday with several songs, as well as regaling all the diners with the lovely melodies of Ireland.
It was one of those islands of calm in a daily world that is increasingly calamitous. (Just noticed that only an "A" changes calm into calamity - the "A" of Alzheimer's?)

Thursday, March 24, 2005
Jack's doctor changed his insulin dosages for breakfast and dinner. Argh. That will cause ten days of grief. However, he finally ordered a series of blood tests to rule out unusual causes of dementia - vitamin B deficiency, metabolic deficiencies, etc. He also ordered an MRI. I am very happy because these are the tests I had wanted done a year ago.

Friday, March 25, 2005
A simple thing like putting the shade back on a night light became a source of frustration. Jack turned it in every direction, including the obviously wrong ones. The man who drew with geometric precision could not put the shade back on a night light.

Saturday, March 26, 2005

Today a haircut became the problem. Not getting the haircut itself, but what currency to use to pay the seventeen dollar tab. A ten dollar bill, a twenty and two singles were laying on the bed. Jack said he wasn't sure that was right. He didn't know it wasn't or how to correct it. That is what kills me! Yesterday and now today.

On a lighter note, the barber would have loved that tip!

Sunday, March 27, 2005

Easter Sunday! Jack was up at 4 a.m., so it was no problem starting out early for the sunrise service at 6:30 a.m. When I looked out the window, it was foggy but one could still see the houses on the other side of the park. We started out slowly and the first mile and a half were okay. But when we turned onto the main road, it was a complete wipeout and whiteout. We couldn't see anything at all. Zip. No street markings, no culverts, no signs, no cars until they were almost on top of us. We could not see the driveway leading into the church parking lot. There is a stoplight further up the road by the grocery store. I knew we could see that a bit before we were at the intersection.

Told Jack that when I said "turn", he should turn. He did. We made a left turn praying no one was coming from the opposite direction at the posted speed of fifty miles per hour.

We couldn't see anything in the lot so Jack drove very slowly in a straight line until we could just see the outline of the stores in the strip mall right in front of us. We turned and used them as a guide to go to a side street that went back toward the church. Once we reached the church, we had to turn and go down that street to pick up Tricia who was dog sitting while a family was on spring break. Then back to the church hugging the curbs which were the only guides that we could see. What an experience!

As I sat in church meditating on the morning, it was so obvious to equate the fog of the morning with the fog of Alzheimer's. Is that what it is like in Jack's brain so often? No wonder that he panics. Is he as anxious each time about getting through the mental fog as we were this morning about getting through nature's fog? I felt so helpless in the fog. Is that how he feels each time Alzheimer's clouds his mind? No wonder he has begun to grow anxious when I am away from him, even when the daily walks take longer because I chat with a neighbor. Does he feel safer when I am there? Have I become his lighthouse in the fog? If so, then I am going to shine as brightly as I can and stay where he can always see me.

Thursday, March 31, 2005
Jack had the MRI this morning. The order for the procedure read: MRI of head. Reason: dementia. After it was over, I asked Jack if the technician had injected anything into his veins. I didn't get a concrete answer. Later on, he said **they** took blood.

This afternoon I received the results of all the blood tests that had been taken. All were within normal range. No surprise.

Friday, April 1, 2005
The endocrinologist called this evening with the results of the MRI. He said it showed some atrophy consistent with memory loss in an older person. He asked if Jack had ever had a stroke. I replied, not to my knowledge. The MRI showed a tiny infarct (area of dead tissue) in the left hemisphere. Overall, there was nothing acute.

The changes in memory were probably the result of Alzheimer's Disease or dementia. He said that there were medicines that would not cure the disease but could slow the progression. Initially, he thought about waiting until the next appointment to talk about it. Then he said that maybe Jack would take the recommendation better from a neurologist if that person told him about the dementia and treatment. I explained that Jack equates dementia with being "crazy" and that any such mention would be counterproductive. He agreed it would be better to focus the referral on the vascular problem.

He asked to speak to Jack and gave him the results concerning the infarct and the name of a neurologist.

Afterward, Jack said it was just more money making. He was fine, knew everything he was doing, and has been fine since he was in Korea. "I don't need a doctor. I've got more faith and people living up there watching over me."

Sunday, April 3, 2005
Daylight savings time. Another change that will cause havoc. These changes never bothered me before. Now that I am trying to make daily life more pleasant by keeping all things the same, it's another wave that rocks the boat.

Last spring, Jack spent a whole evening trying to adjust the time on his glucometer. I finally did it for him. Ditto in the fall. Today, he did not recognize the time as being incorrect. I will change it when he is outside or sleeping.

Tuesday, April 5, 2005
Ever since the endocrinologist spoke with him on Friday, Jack keeps saying that he was told his stomach was moved over. He says he isn't going to have anybody try cutting him to move things around.

Two weeks ago, he was given a medication to control blood pressure and it has been upsetting his stomach. I think he has twisted together what he was told with the upset stomach and it has become one in his mind.

Today he stopped taking the new medication and says he feels better. It was a beautiful day in the seventies and he spent it clearing out the gutters. Still knowing how to do that task is a good strong memory, a plus.

Tonight he showed me a postcard he had filled out and asked me if the address looked right. The zip code was missing. He said, "I don't know what that is."

Thursday, April 7, 2005

Another glitch, more serious than some. When measuring out his insulin dosage, Jack is unsure where the plunger should stop for the correct units. I made a big drawing of two syringes and marked off the stopping point for the morning units on one syringe and on the other syringe the stopping point for the evening injection. Will he get mixed up as to which one is the morning one and which one is the evening one?

I really have no idea how much insulin he has been taking each time since he no longer marks the dosage down on the chart. I wish he would allow me to be with him when he takes his readings and injects insulin. Any attempt to do so on my part is forcefully resisted on his part.

I understand that he is trying to hang on to his independence in every way possible. I respect that. It breaks my heart each time I see a little bit more of it fade away. He has always been fiercely independent. How hard this must be for him. If he understood why I want to do the things for him that he has done for himself, he would be accepting. But if he understood why, there would be no reason to be doing them because his mind would still be intact.

Now that warmer weather is here and there is much for him to do outside, it will be easier to check the glucometer readings, the number of syringes used and how fast the vial of insulin is being depleted without being caught.

THEY LIVED AT OUR HOUSE

Monday, April 11, 2005

Our refund check came from the IRS. In the envelope was a card offering a US Mint 2005 Silver Dollar that could be ordered. It confused Jack. He thought we had to fill the form out and send it back with the refund check. He didn't recognize it as advertising. Once again, the guy who spent his career as an artist in advertising and marketing and designed thousands of ad pieces could not recognize one!

Wednesday, April 13, 2005

The outdoor work is really more than Jack can handle physically. After the winter, there is so much clean up to do in the yard and front lawn. A neighbor gave me the name of a landscaper she uses. He came today at 11:30 a.m. and worked until 5 o'clock. His men did an excellent job of removing the old bushes by the garage, raking up the old leaves and winter debris and aerating the lawn for spring.

Friday, April 15, 2005

I was just starting to fix dinner when the phone rang. LaVerne's voice was panicky. Lately, that is not too unusual.

"I'm done for. It's over. I went to the store and ..." (She paused and my heart was in my mouth. I thought she was going to say she had a car accident.

"...my purse was stolen. Everything is gone. My driver's license, my glasses, everything."

I asked, "Did you call the police?"

"No. I didn't know it was missing until I got home. I had my keys in my hand and got home and went into the house." The more she rambled on, the sketchier it became. Didn't actually see anyone taking it. She didn't call the police because it is vague to her. There was a vague reference to a young girl grabbing her groceries and the cashier saying, "Leave them alone, they are not yours."

She went back to the store, but the purse wasn't there. It was a mystery how it all happened. She said she called her sister, who was attending church. Then she launched into a tirade about the church, and hating God and hating everybody and how close she has come to committing suicide. She hates this damn disease.

Slowly I talked to her and calmed her down and tried to get more information about the purse. She said she searched her house and car. It was hard to see without her regular glasses. She was wearing sunglasses. (Her house is always dark, because she won't use anything brighter than a 40-watt bulb for ambiance – and frugality.)

Calmly suggested that she have something to eat or go and walk around her yard. It would help her clear her mind and try to remember. She hung up.

After dinner, I called her back. The purse was still nowhere to be found and her credit card was in it. She was angry with her sister for telling her she needed to carry her credit card in her purse. I know that was done because LaVerne never has much money in her purse in case of an emergency.

Then she said, "Well, I know I didn't have a driver's license but I wanted ice cream so I went and got some." And she kept on talking. I was intrigued. When she finished talking, I asked her where she had gotten the ice cream. She named another grocery store.

To test her, I asked "What kind?"

She said she always get - paused and looked in the fridge - light French Silk. She said that when she went to pay for it, it was over $9 and that was too much and the cashier said that's because it is not Buy One Get One Free. So LaVerne said she would only take one and she wanted a refund.

I asked her, "Where did you get the money to pay for the ice cream?" It stunned her and she couldn't answer. Also asked her what she did with the money that was refunded. Again, she couldn't answer.

As we were talking, Lee came. Later that evening, Laverne called me back. The purse had been found.

Called Lee for details. When she arrived at LaVerne's, she was concerned about the credit card and helped LaVerne call the company. The customer service rep promptly canceled the card and said the company would replace it with a new number. It sounded like there were quite a few words exchanged between the two sisters.

Afterward she was walking through the foyer on her way to the front door. There is a three-foot statue of the mythical god Pan in the foyer. There was the purse hanging around his neck.

Lee said to LaVerne, "I found your purse."

LaVerne shouted back, "Don't bother me with that. I've got to find my purse."

"LaVerne, I FOUND it!"

Lee said she wished that she had gone there while it was still light. She might have seen the purse then and averted the crisis. But it seemed like there was a crisis everyday and she was tired of missing Mass, oftentimes over little nothings.

She added that after the purse was found, LaVerne insisted on calling the credit card company to get her old number back, an impossibility as we all know.

Thursday, April 21, 2005

Writing checks is more and more of an issue, but Jack avoids all my suggestions to help. He is fine, he says.

Today, his comprehension slipped even further. He was unsure of how to record a deposit in the checkbook transactions record and said "**They** won't know what to do with this." I explained that we are the only ones who see the recorder, not the bank, as he is thinking.

Fortunately, the fact that we have shared the responsibility of the checkbook and the budget book is a great blessing. He always made the entries and I always balanced the checkbook against the statement and added up the columns in the budget book. That has given me access to both without diminishing his need to keep as many tasks as he can. Whatever is amiss can be cleared up at the end of the month.

I know what bills need to be paid. A while back, I suggested to Jack that he write them out. I would seal them and put stamps on since the stamps are always on my desk and it would save him the bother of getting them. He did not object. It gives me an opportunity to make sure the checks are written out correctly and the bills are paid on time. Of course, a new glitch always shows up. A couple of times recently, he has not used the checks in the checkbook but taken ones off the top of pads of checks waiting for future use.

As long as the bills are paid on time and nothing really dastardly is occurring, I am content.

Saturday, April 30, 2005

All week long, Jack has been trying to get the lawnmower to work. It was fully charged and gas and oil were put into it last week after he put a new blade on it. The mower started up and he cut a little of the grass. Then, he stopped it because he thought the blade was making noise. Since then he cannot get it started. He has spent every evening reading the thin manual that came with it. He's read it over and over and over. He has also been reading the manual for the old lawnmower which just adds to his confusion.

It is interesting that he did not have a problem doing the mechanical work of replacing the blade, something he has done for years. The lawnmower is only two years old, so it was purchased when memory problems were already occurring. This may be why the manual for it seems foreign to him and he keeps referring to the old one.

Suggested to Jack that we would have the lawn taken care of by the guy who did such a good job in cleaning up the yard. To my relief, he agreed. He is stymied about the mower. How hard it must be to try solving a problem, when all the pieces of information you need won't stay in your short-term memory.

Saturday, May 7, 2005
Jack and I started painting the overhang along the garage. He is still good on ladders. Getting up and down is harder as he ages but doable.

We are just going to do the areas and windows that really need painting. Let the rest of it go. Jack really can't tackle the whole job anymore, not only physically but also mentally. It is hard for him to plan it out. I'm content to get done what really needs doing and leave the rest for the future. We will probably have painters do it in a few years.

Jack wanted to do this by himself this year. I thought, okay, we'll give it a try. His painting skills are still intact, no skipped spots, no sloppy drips. What is hard for him is thinking the job through. The tools he needs, the paint, the ladder,

Another facet of his life that is fading away. How many more will evaporate until he is left sitting and staring unseeingly into space. The Jack I knew would never want this. Please, God, don't let it come to that, for his sake.

Wednesday, May 11, 2005
After dinner, Jack started talking about Korea and his service there in the Army. This was the very first time he had ever shown so much emotion when talking about it. He choked up and had a hard time going on while relating how a soldier

who was his friend was accidentally but fatally shot by another soldier in the trenches. I never saw tears roll down his cheeks like that.

Only rarely has he spoken about his time in the front lines. And briefly at that. He has always been somber and terse when relating stories of the fighting and hardships. He is a very private person and, until today, always kept his personal emotions under control.

This is a new side of his personality I've never seen before.

Tuesday, May 24, 2005

One of the top wheels on the patio screen door is sunken in and not running right. Jack said he could get a new wheel and went to the hardware store to get one. This evening he took the door off to fix it while Tricia and I went for a walk.

When we returned, he had already taken the wheel off the door. But it was a good wheel from the bottom of the door, not the defective one from the top. When I mentioned this to him, there was the usual outburst of frustration.

He did not comprehend what was wrong because he was having a hard time figuring out which side of the door is the outside and which is the inside, which is the top and which is the bottom. He has also forgotten how to put the door back into the track. Many attempts to reinstall the door in its track made a mess of the perfect paint job done on the patio door frame the other day. These are all things he knew so readily and I didn't. Now I am trying to learn how things work so I can be helpful even when my help isn't wanted.

The Lord always answers our prayers. Tonight I was desperately needing someone with whom I could mentally share something lighthearted. After the tumult of the evening, I thought I would read for a few minutes to refresh my mind. Just grabbed for a book and picked up one on Alzheimers. Great!

That was the last thing I needed to read but I was desperate. I flipped to the section on help for caregivers and there was my answer. Listings of websites for humor. Just had a minute to try one. Now I know where to go when I need a little laugh pin to prick the stress balloon and let out just enough so it doesn't burst. This is good. Thank you, God, for guiding my hand.

Thursday, May 26, 2005
On Monday, LaVerne worked outside in the yard all day. When she came into the house, she couldn't find her regular eyeglasses. She went outside and started looking all over for them including the little creek behind her house. Her neighbor helped her look and kept saying "I don't think they are here, LaVerne. I saw you outside all day long and you had your sunglasses on."

Yesterday, she called Lee who came over to help her search the house. She brought two pairs of backup glasses for LaVerne to use until she found her own or had a new pair made. As she was getting out of the car, Lee handed them to LaVerne, telling her, *"Be sure not to lose these. I want them back."* LaVerne promptly put the eyeglasses on the grass and started picking up more sticks.

After searching the house fruitlessly, LaVerne was taken to the optical shop to order a new pair of glasses. When they returned, Lee mentioned that they had eaten out on Sunday. Maybe the eyeglasses had been left at the restaurant.

Today, LaVerne called me and said that she had gone to the restaurant. She said she asked if they had her glasses. The man gave her a box of unclaimed glasses to go through. She said that her glasses weren't in the box. But she didn't like the ones she was wearing. She found a nice pair in the box that she liked better. So she put the ones she had on (Lee's backups) in the box and took the pair she liked!

Friday, May 27, 2005

Lee took LaVerne to pick up her eyeglasses. Then they stopped at a deli to have lunch. LaVerne was constantly fiddling with her glasses.

"Why do I have these glasses?"

"You lost your old ones."

"Don't I have another pair of glasses?"

"Those glasses are mine."

"Where are the dark glasses?"

"You were wearing your sunglasses because you lost your other ones."

"Are these sunglasses new ones?"

"No, the sunglasses are old ones. You have the new glasses on."

"I don't understand. These glasses don't look like mine."

"The glasses you were wearing earlier aren't yours. You picked them out of the box at the restaurant when the man took you into the room and gave you the box."

"He didn't take me into a room! The man said the glasses are outside on the grass. And that's where they were laying on the grass outside the door."

This is a good example of what and how the brain afflicted with dementia works. LaVerne had a memory of being at the restaurant asking about her glasses. She had a memory of taking the spare pairs of eyeglasses and putting them on the grass. Everything in between might be missing. So she just puts the two together. Makes sense to her.

Tuesday, June 7, 2005

A day of grace! This evening I walked into the bedroom and saw that, once again, Jack had all the pads of new checks spread out on the bed. He said he was looking for a ticket to write out for the gas bill. I pulled the checkbook out from the dresser drawer and showed him the next check to be written. He said that it didn't look right to him. Futilely, he kept trying to put the pads of new checks in numerical order.

Holding my breath, I mentioned to him that I knew he had so much to do and I wanted to help. If he wanted, I would write out all the checks so he wouldn't have to do it. And just like that, he said, "Okay."

Okay! No agitation. No frustration. He seemed relieved. He promptly picked up the boxes of new checks and started putting them in my hands. He pulled out the pads of deposit slips and put them in my hands. He gave me the transaction folders. And he lost no time in digging in the back of the closet and giving me a metal box with every canceled check he had written since May 1, 1964!

I am so grateful that God resolved this ongoing problem without any upset and before things got too far out of hand. God is good.

Thursday, June 9, 2005

Several months ago we found out that the State of Illinois was holding unclaimed property for Jack. The check came today covering the value of a policy his mother took out over sixty years ago. It was probably one of those five-hundred dollar ones. An insurance man with a huge ledger under his arm would come to the house every week to collect five or ten cents.

When Jack receives a check now, he reads everything on it. When I asked him what the amount was, he gave me the date, the check number, the bank number, and everything else but the amount.

He became very concerned that he needed two people to witness his signature when he signed the check. I reassured him that that was only for people who couldn't write their name and had to sign it with an "x". When he went to the bank to cash the check, he insisted I go with him (was going to, anyway) because **they** would give him a hassle. The teller never batted an eyelash when she made the transaction.

Wednesday, June 15, 2005

The past few days have been very difficult. Jack has not been on friendly terms with his glucometer. "**They** don't know what **they** are doing. It's a piece of junk."

Tricia was asking her dad where he wanted to go for dinner on Father's Day. Afterward, he asked me in all seriousness, "Did she say next Sunday is my birthday?"

This disease is so depressing for people around the person afflicted. It is cruel to rob one of their memory and capability, bit by bit by bit.

My dear friend, Rose, sent me *The Notebook* by Nicholas Sparks. It's a novel about a couple who have been together for forty-nine years and the effects of Alzheimer's on their lives. I can't put it down. I keep reading snatches of it every chance I have. Terrific story, topnotch writing, and so true.

Thursday, June 16, 2005

After being so depressed yesterday, the liturgy readings from Isaiah this morning were about turning darkness into light, a spiritual hug, when all the light in our lives is being eclipsed by the darkness of this disease.

Then one of my sisters called and said she and her husband were driving out. We went out for lunch and had a relaxing time and good conversation.

Jack told me beforehand that he wanted to pay for lunch and would use his credit card because it would be easier. I knew he did not want to go through the hassle of figuring out the money. It was a smart thought.

When the waitress brought the credit card receipt he gave her cash and said it was the tip. She smiled and said, "Thank you!" He signed the receipt and gave it back to her.
This evening he said, "I gave her (the waitress) five dollars. I think that was all right."
I asked, "A five-dollar tip?"
He said, "Yes, five and five and five and five" (as he counted out four fingers). One for each of us."
He certainly made that waitress' day, a twenty-dollar tip on a forty-five dollar lunch bill.
It was worth it to see him happy and pleased with himself for a change.
It was a very good day.

Thursday, June 23, 2005
The new file cabinet I ordered for Jack as a Father's Day gift arrived today. The key and one screw are missing. The screw is no problem. There are a hundred baby food jars in the basement with nuts and bolts and screws and nails of every type and size.

We spent an hour working on it. Me holding the flashlight so he could see inside the drawer and he trying to put the handles and label holder on. Finally, he gave up and said he would do it in the morning. I asked if I could fiddle with it. He said, "**They** sent you a piece of junk and you won't get anywhere with it." I finished it off within a few minutes. Something he would have been able to do if it weren't for this horrible disease. Instead I'm reminding him that the handle should be screwed on to the outside of the drawer, not the inside.

The guy who put together bikes and trikes and jungle gyms and shelving units and innumerable other items, who designed and built all of the display units we used for the shows, spent a frustrating hour trying to follow instructions for attaching two handles to a file cabinet, finally concluding that **they** didn't know what **they** were doing. **They** wrote the instructions wrong.

However, he still can put in light bulbs and filters and put air in the tires and some other things, so I am thankful that there are still tasks he can do so he feels useful and needed. That is the hardest part of dealing with this disease, trying to help or even takeover some activities when it becomes difficult or impossible for him to do them. And to do it in such a way that it doesn't diminish his self-esteem.

These past two years, especially, have been a learning experience. All the knowledge I gained in reading about and dealing with the developmental problems that Tricia and her classmates had in school is now being put to good use. I have learned that it really is no different. Whether the memory deficit is in the very young child or in the aging adult, the coping mechanisms should be the same. The only difference to keep in mind is that the young child does not know what he or she is missing and needs to be taught in an affirmative manner. The adult who is losing memory has experienced what is now missing and is inwardly frantic about losing what they still have.

Both need to live in environments that are as calm as can be, are structured, are not filled with too many changes, and are positive.

Correcting mistakes in a negative fashion is as detrimental to the adult as it is to the child. Constantly saying, "No, this is the correct word or name" or "that's not how it happened" is demeaning to the person and ultimately self-defeating to the caregiver because it usually irritates the person being corrected. Of course, serious situations such as using machinery or proper dosages of medicine need correction.

Loved ones close to the person with memory loss often keep correcting them hoping to make the person better than they can be. In the long run, whether Abraham Lincoln was the 12th president or the 30th or whether Aunt Mabel or Aunt Clara ate the whole jar of pickles doesn't matter. The only fact that matters is loving that person as they are, not as one would like them to be.

Jack does best in familiar surroundings and situations and routines. When the days unfold with no new crisis, nothing breaks or stops working, the mail doesn't bring communications he can't understand, he is able to do one thing at a time with nothing else interfering, and he isn't asked to do something new, life is rather harmonious. I am happy and content to try and make every day like that for him.

Friday, June 24, 2005
There has been some self-serving in getting the new file cabinet for Jack. I knew that Jack would have incentive to go through all the files in order to move them from the old cabinet to the new one. And I would offer to help.

Ever since the fiasco with the credit card, he has been overly concerned that he has not been getting a credit card statement and the bills are piling up and we are going to owe thousands of dollars when it finally comes. He is not convinced that a statement has come every month and everything is up to date. What he does have is an ever-growing file of grocery store receipts. I have asked to see the statements to match them up with the receipts, to no avail. The response always is "I'm telling you **they** haven't billed this and when **they** send it, it's going to be thousands of dollars."

Today, as we (yes, I was allowed to help) were transferring files, I said that, if he wanted, I'd straighten up the huge file with all the receipts hanging out of it. There were statements from 2003 and 2004 with receipts stuffed into each envelope. The statements for 2005 had no envelopes full of receipts. I asked why the receipts weren't with the statements. He said he was still waiting for a statement for the receipts that weren't in envelopes.

I asked Jack to pick out a receipt and tell me the date and the total, which he did. I found it on one of the statements and showed him that it had been paid. We did another. Then another. We went through all the receipts until only the latest two were not in an envelope. He looked at those two receipts and said, "Well, **they** finally came to their senses!" He started moving other files. And that was that.

Tuesday, June 28, 2005

Calendars are now incomprehensible to Jack. Since there are five Sundays in July, the last Sunday square is divided 24/31. It is beyond Jack's understanding. It does not make any sense to him. The guy who designed and coordinated the yearly calendar programs for his company's offices, factories and affiliates, now looks at a calendar as if he had never seen one before.

Friday, July 1, 2005

The doctor asked Jack quite a few questions about his present readings, insulin doses, what he did in the past, his army service in Korea, his education. He told Jack that his long-term memory was very good, but he needed help with the short-term memory. He asked Jack if he would see a neurologist. Jack said, "Yes." I wonder if he actually will.

As usual, we stopped for lunch on our way home and it was a pleasant time. I relish these moments because they are few and far between.

Sunday, July 3, 2005

No surprise, Jack is backing off from seeing a neurologist. "That guy doesn't know what he's talking about. There's nothing wrong with me. I've been going along fine for years. **They** are the ones who need help. **They** are not going to do anything to me. I know what I am doing. I'd be dead already if I had gone along with **them**."

Then, out of the clear blue, he said, "Remember the other night at dinner when you said you would fix rolls and you didn't. You forget, too."

I chuckled to hear him say that. This was saving face. There's still a lot of spunk there. That's good.

Monday, July 4, 2005

Jack showed me the card for his next appointment with the endocrinologist. It read: "Tues. 10/04/05 11:15 a.m." It didn't make any sense to him. Not even when I explained that October was the tenth month of the year. None of it means anything to him any more.

We have been walking together in the evening. It feels so good to be together quietly.

Friday, July 15, 2005

A lighter day. In the morning we went to the riverboat casino. It is one of the few pleasures Jack still enjoys, even though it, too, is getting confusing. We don't go very often but when we do we go in the morning when there are fewer patrons. We stay together and I enjoy the pleasure he gets from pulling that handle.

And he always is lucky. He was last year and he was today. He put one coin into a fifty-cent slot machine and won $450 on that one play with a special symbol that paid out nine times the normal jackpot. He won some small jackpots and cashed in $625.

We stopped at a hamburger shop for lunch. I teased him about winning megabucks and only being able to afford burgers.

Wednesday, July 20, 2005

This morning Jack asked me if today was Wednesday. Yes. "Well, isn't it your birthday or something?"

How it hurts and I want to cry during the tirades when he emphatically insists that he is fine, his mind is fine, and then he asks questions like this. The man who made me the envy of all my friends because he never missed any occasion: birthday, anniversary, Valentines, St. Patrick's Day, Easter, Mother's Day, Sweetest Day, Christmas. He delighted in remembering them all.

On Mother's Day in one of the years before Tricia was born, he gifted me with flowers for potential.

Sunday, July 31, 2005

Tricia was out for the day. Jack and I went to the local restaurant for a late lunch/early dinner. It's been hot and I had a taste for their crab salad sandwich. Apparently so did everyone else because there wasn't any left.

While we were eating, the waitresses were sitting at a large round table across from our booth. It was mid afternoon and the restaurant wasn't busy. They were either on break eating their own lunches or they were rolling flatware into napkins for the dinner crowd. All the while they were enjoying each other's company.

One of the waitresses is attending classes to earn a degree in nursing. This led to talk about the nursing home across the street, the different levels of nursing care, and eventually dementia and Alzheimer's Disease.

The woman earning her degree said dementia was the precursor of Alzheimer's. Dementia was short-term memory loss. Alzheimer's Disease encompassed significant decline and personality changes. She explained that her grandmother had had Alzheimer's. As she put it "my grandmother was a petite, gentle woman who went to Mass eight days a week and had religious articles all over her house. As the disease progressed, when you entered her bedroom you would have thought she was the Godfather by her actions and what came out of her mouth."

How true. The agitation and the clenched fists and arms waving about. That's not Jack. It's another person.

Trying to do things or fix things. Not quite being able to remember how to. Sort of like my sewing a sleeve to a neckline instead of to the armhole, and when told it is wrong, not seeing or understanding that it is or where it should belong. Not saying "Oh, for Pete's sake, whatever made me do that." Instead, getting agitated but not quite knowing why.

Monday, August 1, 2005

At 1 a.m., Tricia called on her cell phone. She had been in a car accident. She reassured me that she is fine. Just a few nicks from flying glass. She said, "The paramedics told me my vital signs were fine. But my stomach is all shook up."

The driver was okay, except for a deep cut on his elbow from the side view mirror. He was bringing her home down Milwaukee Avenue in an area that's under road construction. An oncoming driver sideswiped the car knocking off the side view mirror which cut the driver's elbow, then flew thru the car and smashed the rear window behind Tricia. She said they had to go to the hospital so her friend could get stitches in his elbow. Then he would drive her home

When she called me they were standing by the side of the road where the accident happened, in the dark, in front of a cemetery waiting for someone to come and jump-start the car's battery. The car lights were on while the police were there and drained the battery. I kept her on the phone until someone came. My mother's imagination was thinking who knows who could stop and take advantage of their predicament in such a dark spot late at night.

All the while I was on the phone Jack wanted to know what was going on. I didn't want to tell him everything. As it was, the facts I did tell him caused a bout of agitation.

He decided he was going to pick her up. Driving in unfamiliar areas in the dark of night with mist on the ground thru road construction, I knew he couldn't do this alone. At the very least, it was a certainty he would get lost. Most likely, he would have an accident, even if it were only going off the road in the mist. But I would not go. There was too much at risk. I needed to keep myself intact to be here for him and for Tricia.

He was angry because I did not want him to drive. "I've been up there before (a few times quite a few years ago in broad daylight and it was a hassle) and I can do it again. You keep thinking that I can't do anything." And so it went for several minutes.

Finally, I suggested that before he goes anywhere, he should check his glucose level. Fortunately, he agreed. The reading was seventy, a bit low. He needed to eat something before he left. We went into the kitchen and I fixed toast and tea. While he was eating, I was successful in getting him to start talking about past job experiences. He calmed down and talked for a long time.

Meanwhile, Tricia called from the hospital in Libertyville. She said she would be home in an hour. She was worried that her dad would be angry with her when she came home. She said her stomach was upset enough. I reassured her that there is no reason for her dad to be upset. It was an accident. She is fine. And so is her friend. That's all her dad and I care about.

When she and her friend pulled into the driveway, dawn was beginning to break. We went out to see how they were. The driver was very apologetic. He felt responsible for her safety. I assured him that he shouldn't apologize. He should be thanked. We were grateful.

The oncoming driver was drunk, crossed over into the wrong lane and had begun to come at their vehicle head on. By swerving to the right, her friend had prevented the accident from becoming a head-on collision with the other driver's truck.

Jack was glad to see that Tricia was okay. She was relieved. The sun was up brightly at 6 a.m., when the three of us finally went to bed.

Monday, August 8, 2005

At lunch, we were listening to news coverage of the death of Peter Jennings, the ABC world news anchor who died of lung cancer. When the reporter noted that Jennings was sixty-seven, Jack said, "That's in my ball park." I asked him what he meant. He replied, "I'm sixty-seven."

He's lost the meaning of age. How horrible not to know how old you are, where you stand in the chronology of age. This is the first time he has actually mentioned his age, or what he thought it is.

How I hate this disease! Anyone who has been afflicted with it has to go straight to heaven. How could justice not be fulfilled? What prison could be worse?

LaVerne called tonight and was all upset. She thought she had missed my birthday. I told her she had not. It is Wednesday.

Tuesday, August 9, 2005

During the last few days, Jack has been uncertain about my birthday. This morning he came home with a big bouquet of red roses. Absolutely beautiful. He did not say Happy Birthday. I wondered if he had gotten them today because we had plans for tomorrow morning.

At dinnertime he kept asking where Tricia was. I told him she wasn't having dinner with us because she had been out with friends and had a big lunch. He said, "She's never around when you want her to be."

After he finished eating, he went down to the basement and brought up a bag which he placed by my chair. I asked if he wanted me to save it until tomorrow. He said, "No."

The birthday card has the most beautiful saying about two people needing each other and it brought tears to my eyes. He was upset because he had written *All May Love,* instead of *My.* It's a good sign that he recognized the mistake!

Tonight LaVerne called again to wish me a Happy Birthday. Reminded her that it was tomorrow.

Wednesday, August 10, 2005

Jack was up at 4 a.m. for 6:30 a.m. Mass. He had had cereal and orange juice before going to bed last night. He was still concerned about the time.

As we drove east to church for a Mass of thanksgiving for reaching sixty-two, the sunrise was gorgeous. Mostly gray clouds but in the east a small break in them with rays of golden light pouring out in every direction. And, even though there had been no rain, to my utter delight, a rainbow!

How I love rainbows. What a sign of hope! Eagerly I look for each and every one and savor the peace that floods my heart each time I see one. All is well in God's world.

At breakfast, the waitress was asking the couple behind us about a man who used to come in every morning with friends. She wondered if he had had a stroke because he seemed out of it the last time he was in. The couple said he has Alzheimer's. They also talked about another man who had been an arbitrator for a well-known company and who now has Alzheimer's. The waitress said that it scared her more than cancer.

The afternoon was filled with congratulatory phone calls and a futile attempt to access e-mail cards on the internet. Frank sent a stunning bouquet of flowers. The plan was to go to dinner between 4:30 and 5 p.m.

Around 4 p.m., I was just signing off the computer and planning to freshen up when Jack walked out of the bedroom all ready to go. He said he had taken a reading and it was 227. I said it was better than a hypoglycemic reaction. He said, "We have to go immediately because I need something to eat." And so we went.

The past few days have been overflowing with continuous confusion related to the glucose readings, insulin dosages, the correct time and day. What fog permeates his brain where morning and evening and night are interchangeable and dates and time and numbers lose their meaning? Personally, I am adamant that God should not allow Alzheimer's Disease in a type 1 insulin-dependent diabetic.

Dinner was very enjoyable. The London broil and salad were excellent. And left just enough room for a delicious slice of apple pie with warm caramel topping.

In the evening I tried again to access the e-mail greeting cards. Got right to the site. Only problem was that the top of the site reads: A greeting from... and the rest of the page is blank. Stared at those blank pages and thought how apropos they were at this point in time. I feel blank. I turned sixty-two today and feel more like eighty, especially mentally.

But as Scarlet O'Hara would say, "Tomorrow's another day."

LaVerne never did call today.

Thursday, August 11, 2005

In late July, during one of her daily calls, LaVerne told me that she had lunch with a good friend of hers who had borrowed a set of my books. LaVerne told me they were in a bag by the front door. I was going to suggest that she put them in the gold box in the back hall where she usually keeps everything she wants to give me. Thought better of it. If she did that and then didn't see the books by the front door, she might panic because she didn't remember putting them in the gold box.

A few days later, LaVerne still called in a panic. She could not find the books. I told her not to worry about them. I didn't need them now. They will turn up somewhere. She, however, went on a massive hunt of the house trying to find them without success.

Tonight her friend called me and asked what was going on with LaVerne. She said LaVerne had called her and was very angry that she still had the books. She told LaVerne that she had brought the books to LaVerne's house and put them by the railing in the foyer. LaVerne replied that the friend had called LaVerne a week earlier and told her that she had the books but was too busy to bring them and LaVerne could come and get them. LaVerne said, "You know I don't know how to get to your house."

I told the friend what I knew about the books. She said that the day the two of them had lunch, LaVerne had told her she had Alzheimer's.

She said her mom had had it. For a long time her mom would buy things and forget where she put them, forget to cook meals, etc. and the family would laugh. They had no idea what it was or how serious it was. She said that when her father was ill in the hospital, he had said, "When I'm better, we have to do something about mom. Something's not right." He never came home. The mom lived with her daughter for five years.

One day a cousin came for a visit with his child. After he left, her mom said, "Who was that nice man?" That's when she knew it was serious. Her mom would often say, "You know, something is happening to me, but I don't know what it is."

Because she worked, she hired caregivers to be with her mom during the day. But her mom was up at all hours of the night and she couldn't keep up. Her mom needed to live in a facility with a secure environment.

Sunday, August 14, 2005

Last year I bought a book called *Into the Shadows* by Robert DeHaan. it describes his wife's journey into Alzheimer's Disease. I started reading it then, but never finished because life intervened. Began rereading it a few weeks ago and found more meaning in it now that months have gone by in our lives. Today, I needed a rest and decided to finish the book during the day between the necessities of life.

Both the author and his wife, Roberta, are well-educated professors with a wide range of accomplishments and interests and a deep religious grounding with a very active membership in the First United Methodist Church of Germantown. Originally, they hailed from Grand Rapids where they met at college. He was taken with her the first day in a geometry class when she correctly named every theory described by the professor while everyone else was scratching their heads.

When he knew for certain that Roberta had Alzheimer's, he decided to return to Grand Rapids to be near his sister and other relatives. Shortly after they moved into their new apartment in Grand Rapids, Roberta began uncontrollable night walking and wandering. That and other issues made Robert realize that he could no longer care for her on his own. She was admitted into assisted living. A few months later she was moved to a secure skilled care unit because of the incessant night wandering.

On the last page of the book was a note from the author dated January 2003 stating that he was planning a second book based on their lives lived apart. He had an independent living apartment in the same complex where she was living.

I decided to see if the second book was published. I googled his name on the internet. It came up with too many leads for hundreds of Robert DeHaan's. So I googled Roberta's name and came up with a smaller list among which was the book I had read. Then I saw one item labeled FUMCOG, which gave a few words about a service for Robert DeHaan.

I clicked on it and found in the In Memoriam column a notice about a memorial service on February 21st for Robert DeHaan who died on January 29, 2005. Condolences could be sent to Roberta DeHaan at Holland House, Breton Park Drive, Grand Rapids, MI. I was stunned. She is still alive, but he is not.

I went to bed with my eyes wide open, contemplating what I read and the course of events. Very unsettling. Finally fell asleep around 3 a.m.

Friday, August 19, 2005

In June when the attempt to get Jack to use the new glucometer was unsuccessful, I prayed for patience. Once again, God worked things out. On the 8th when Jack couldn't get a reading because he was unwittingly diluting his blood sample with alcohol, I used the new meter and got a quick reading.

Afterward, I suggested that we continue to use the new meter. He agreed. For ten days now, there has been no resistance. I handle the new meter so there are no problems with what button to press. Slowly, I have also started to get the lancet and alcohol swab ready and now the syringe. There have been no objections, so I try to be there each time until it becomes normal for me to be there. Now I know whether Jack took insulin and how much.

What was taking fifteen or more minutes on good days is now back down to the five minutes it used to be for many years. I no longer have to wonder about whether insulin was taken, when, and how much. Praise the Lord! What a relief.

Thursday, August 25, 2005

As we were walking into the kitchen this morning, Jack asked, "Where is Mother?"

Again, as he sat down, he asked, "Where is Mother?"

Then he said, "She passed on, didn't she?"
"Yes."
"I can't seem to get it straight in my mind. Where's Mother? ... She passed on, didn't she?"
"Yes, a long time ago."
"Well, where have you been?"
"Right here."
"I don't see her or you. Were you working?"
"No. I've always been at home."
"I don't see you here."
No reply from me.
"Well, where have you been sleeping?"
"Right next to you."
"I can't see you here."
"You and Tricia and I moved here together."
"No one else was here? Mother was never here?"
"No."
"She passed on?"
"Yes."
"I know I was working, but I don't see Mother."
"Where were you working?" (Trying to figure out where in the past his mind was.)
"At the electric company."
"Do you remember moving here?"
"Yes, but I don't remember you being here."
"I was."
"Was Dad ever here?"
"No, he wasn't. He passed on and that's why we moved here."
"He never lived here? But it seems like he's living here and working here but when I come home from work, he's never here."
"He never lived here."
"He passed on?"

"Yes, he and your Mother lived with us in our old house. Your Mother passed on a long time ago. When your Father passed on, you wanted to move..."

"I know but it seems so strange."

He sat for quite a while with an open, puzzled look on his face, trying to get his thoughts to make sense. Then he said,

"It's only us here."

"Yes, you and Tricia and me."

"Sometimes when I wake up, I think we have to go to church, but...." he trailed off.

"Not today. It's Thursday."

"It's so confusing. I can't get it straight in my mind."

And so the conversation went on and on for well over half an hour.

Friday, September 2, 2005

Yesterday evening, Jack was disturbed again about taking his pension check to the local bank. He wanted cash but couldn't figure out how to do it. He kept saying "**They'll** mess it up. It can't be done." I asked him how much cash he needed. He couldn't tell me if he needs fives, tens or twenties. Just kept saying "It can't be done. I'm going to have a problem when I get there. **They** screwed me up before. **They** kept giving me a slip of paper when I wanted cash."

Last time, Jack had a check for sixty-four dollars. He filled out a deposit slip, when he wanted to cash the check. It confused the teller. She deposited the money and gave him a receipt.

This morning I had several bank transactions to make on my business and personal accounts and asked Jack if he wanted me to do his. He said, "Yes, but **they** are going to give you a big problem." Figured out how many bills to ask for from fives to fifties, since I don't know what he needs. He seemed perplexed at how easily it worked.

On the way home we stopped for gas. The station was out. There were no deliveries because of Hurricane Katrina. Now Jack is convinced that we won't be able to get regular gas, anymore. **They** won't sell it so they can make money on higher priced gas.

Tuesday, September 6, 2005
The appointment with the ophthalmologist is next Monday. Jack has been agitated about it. "He's not doing anything to my eyes." In May, he was told that the cataract on the left eye was hindering his vision and could be removed in the fall. When I mention that he had the right eye done three years ago, he insists that he never had anything done to his eyes. Yet, he found the black case which he was given three years ago with all the old drops, etc. He started to look at the instruction sheet and became very upset. It mentioned that he couldn't drive for twenty-four hours and should have someone come with him to drive him home. That's what I did three years ago. He doesn't believe it.

He has a real fear about my driving. He doesn't want me to drive at all. Just mentioning it causes agitation. He is always worried that I will have an accident. At first, I thought that he was worried about losing his independence and self worth. If I do all the driving, then is he needed? Lately I am convinced that the fear that is at the source is not the fear of losing his independence. Rather, he is afraid that if something happens to me and I am not here, what would happen to him? How would he cope?

Thursday, September 8, 2005
The vehicle emission test notice for the '85 Chevy came in the mail today. Jack said **they** won't pass "a thirty-nine year-old car". I said, "It's twenty years old." He insists it is older than

that. All day long he has been looking at the postcard and considering it a big threat because it states that if you don't get the car tested and fixed to pass the emissions test, your license could be suspended. That's all he needed to read!

Saturday, September 10, 2005

Jack was up early in the morning. When I asked why, he said he had to work on the Chevy so it would look good when we went for the emissions test. After breakfast, he pulled out his cloths and a pail and the car polish. He went into the garage to pull the car onto the driveway to work on it. He turned the key in the ignition, nothing happened. He tried again and again. The car would not start.

I suggested that maybe it was time to part with the car. The same suggestion in January when it needed a new battery was not well received. Now he was in agreement. In the evening I found the phone number of a car parts company that would buy old cars.

Sunday, September 11, 2005

After lunch Jack went to get everything out of the glove compartment and trunk. Called to see if anyone might be there on a Sunday, since that's the day guys have to work on their old cars and are looking for parts. They were open and gave me the information I needed. Made an appointment for Tuesday, the 13th. Jack is content to know it can be done.

God is answering my prayers. Slowly, He is eliminating the hurdles that do or will make life more difficult. He took care of the problems with the checkbook, the insulin and glucose readings, now the extra car. I know that eventually I will have to do all of the driving. It will be so much easier for me not to have to slide the car in and out of a confined space. Both cars are full size models. This will also be a good yearly savings: no repairs, gas, oil, insurance, license, sticker, etc. Thank You, God!

Tuesday, September 13, 2005

All weekend long Jack has been obsessing about how the car couldn't be moved out of the garage because there was no power and the wheels were frozen. All weekend long. He was up at 3 a.m. this morning eating breakfast so he'd be dressed and ready.

About 8 a.m. this morning a wiry fellow rang the doorbell, handed me the morning paper and asked, "Is the coffeepot on?" He told Jack he'd been picking up cars for thirty years and there never was one he couldn't get. Very personable guy who knew exactly how to maneuver his truck. He had the car out of the garage and was gone in twenty minutes. We had signed over the title and received a token payment.

After he left, I mentioned that I would love to paint the garage walls. The fifty shades of dust and smudge have been bugging me for years. We started moving everything. Jack actually threw some old things out and by late afternoon we had everything stacked near the center on one side.

Tuesday, September 20, 2005

The past week has been spent working in the garage. The walls and woodwork needed to be washed and double-coated with paint. We teamed up as usual with Jack doing the ladder work on the upper walls and me doing the windows and lower regions. He still has his 'high wire' abilities and it doesn't faze him.

Everything was paced so we wouldn't get overtired. The weather was sunny but not hot. More things were carried out to the curb for pickup. Not as many as I had hoped, but it is a start.

The whole garage looks brighter, cheerier and neater. It has been a very good week.

Saturday, October 1, 2005

How will the day evolve? It has been difficult to gauge how much Jack realizes that today is our 39th wedding anniversary.

It is early morning with the dew glistening on the emerald grass like so many diamonds. Jack is still asleep. No repeat of our yearly attendance at 6:30 a.m. Mass in thanksgiving. If I had mentioned it, he would have been up at 3 a.m., so we wouldn't be late. It is too tiring for both of us. The Lord knows my heart. I am doing what I can.

And, yes, as I think about it, I am very thankful for all these years we have had together. Sometimes, people will ask, "If you knew what was going to happen, would you have still married him?" Without a doubt. I marvel that they would even ask the question. The vow was for better or worse, in sickness and in health, 'til death do us part. I don't know what other people feel when they say their marriage vows, but I meant every word and I know so did Jack.

When Jack brought up the subject of his diabetes, early in our dating, he was concerned about its effect on his longevity. I stated then that I would rather spend six months with him than a lifetime with someone else. I meant it then. I still do.

It is now late evening and I no longer have to wonder how the day unfolded. It was a good day, rather calm. We had talked about the upcoming anniversary during the week, so it had been brought to Jack's attention.

He never thought of a card or flowers or candy, totally not Jack. He wasn't sure why I was giving him a card or gift. I wonder if in his mind he thinks it is vaguely something to do with me, as he said a week ago, and doesn't involve him. In the past year, the something has become even more vague.

THEY LIVED AT OUR HOUSE

Saturday, October 8, 2005

Life is bittersweet. The bitter is that all the abstracts - date, time, month, year – are fading into the shadows so rapidly that Jack rarely sees them.

The sweet is a delectable dinner we had tonight courtesy of our dear next door neighbors who gave us a gift certificate to a seafood house for our anniversary. We had a cozy booth for two, set off by itself with a light bright enough to please Jack (the candlelight dinners bit the dust a long time ago). Rock lobster tails perfectly done, veggies, a salad with warm cheddar rolls and cheesecake and we were in seventh heaven. It was a week later, but it was the perfect anniversary celebration. A time to remember.

Sunday, October 9, 2005

All week long I have been trying to read snatches of a new book I bought last Saturday in the church gift shop. It's entitled *"A Long Good Night - My Father's Journey into Alzheimer's* by Daphne Simpkin. Tonight I decided to use one of Jack's old habits (he was a bathroom reader). I went into the powder room just to read. Maybe I could finish the book without interruption.

The father lost all functions for the most part. However, it is so individual a disease that he didn't become bedridden or totally unable to walk by forgetting how for any great length of time. The writer had been very truthful about the situation. So much hit home. So much may still be to come.

The chapter which began with her wondering what it would be like to be in jail really hit home. She knew that it wouldn't take much for someone to translate her father's bruises from constantly losing his balance and falling, into parental abuse by a daughter. She said that if someone came to the house at a time when her father needed a shave and he had just soiled his clothes, it was an open and shut case.

The same thoughts crossed my mind before Jack would allow me to help him with his readings and insulin intake. If he accidentally overdosed, would it look suspicious? Especially, if someone thought that the dementia could give me reason to take the easy way out? How I can empathize with the feelings she had at the time.

There are horrible diseases from which people suffer and their pain and that of their loved ones cannot be taken lightly. But I can't think of any disease that is as insidious, devastating, and, yes, evil. It steals away a person's abilities, capabilities, thoughts, personality bit by bit in a most painful way both for the person and those who love her or him.

And even more cruelly, every once in a while the disease allows a moment when the losses seem to be erased and the person briefly appears to be and act 'like their old self'. And the loved one rejoices, all the while knowing that the moment won't last and the curtain will descend and the pain will be even worse.

Thursday, October 13, 2005

They were at our house again today. The vials of eye drops and insulin were all mixed up in the wrong boxes. All were in the fridge when two should have been left on the dresser. "**They** have been messing around here again. I always put the drops in the right place. It's my eyes. I've been putting drops in my eyes since before you were born."

In the afternoon Jack spent a considerable amount of time in the basement. When he came up, he said he "couldn't find what he was looking for. **They** keep putting all those books on my storage shelf."

He grew agitated because he was having a difficult time while taking his reading and insulin before dinner. I see the frustration, but if I try to do more than he will allow, it only causes the agitation to become greater. He is fighting for his independence. It is so much easier to deal with these explosions, painful as they are, knowing that they are always beyond his control. I keep remembering who he *was* and love him all the more because he is so afflicted.

Afflicted. I've always associated that word with the Bible and days of yore. People were afflicted with leprosy or palsy. Modern people have problems or illnesses which they present to specialists for treatment. The word rolled off the tip of my pen before I knew what was happening. Alzheimer's is an affliction that is always present. But whether the reality is so obvious you can't miss it, or so subtle you only feel it, it is inexorably invading every nook and cranny of daily life.

Sunday, October 16, 2005

October seems to be the defining month as far as Jack's decline. It was two years ago in October that I knew for sure that he had Alzheimer's as I caught myself giving him the answer to a question that I would give to a little child.

For the past several days, Jack has been poring over the catalogs sitting by the drawing board in his workroom. This afternoon, he went into the bedroom and closed the door. Always a sure sign that he is going to make a phone call. A check of the telephone proved correct. The in-use light gleamed red.

A half hour later, a neighbor stopped by for our daily walk. The bedroom door was still shut preventing me from getting sunglasses and the keys from my purse. I decided to go without. Scribbled a note for Jack so he wouldn't worry when he was finished using the phone.

As we were ready to leave, Jack called to me. He said a fellow on the phone wanted to talk to his wife. When I picked up the phone, the fellow asked if I was Stephanie Heavey (both our names are on the company's catalogs to avoid duplicates). He said his name was Larry and he was a supervisor.

He asked, "Should your husband be ordering on the phone? We've been on the phone for half an hour for one order. Is he all right?"

I replied, "Yes, I understand." Jack was standing next to me with an upset look on his face.

Larry proceeded to tell me that Jack had ordered an item. He could not tell me what it was. It would be sent in a box with a label that reads 'Do Not Open Until Xmas'. The box should arrive by October 25th. He verified that the shipping address was the same as the address to which the credit card bills are sent. I asked for the Order Confirmation number.

Jack was upset, but not agitated, having someone ask for me. He said he called once to place the order and had a woman whom he couldn't understand. She kept asking him something and when he said he couldn't figure out what she wanted, she hung up on him. He said he told them he'd been ordering from them for years and never had a problem They even delivered something to him when he was fishing!? (That's a new one.) But he didn't know what was going on. **They** didn't seem to know what **they** were doing.

How humiliating it is for him! And how my heart breaks for him. The only grace is that he does not realize the truth. Or, if he does, he is a master at pretending that he doesn't. But Jack never pretends. He is what he is. And if he truly doesn't realize what is happening, then my heart is filled with thanks to God for not giving him that pain. And, as much as is humanly possible, I am dedicated to protecting him from any further humiliation and distress.

Later in the afternoon, Jack suggested ordering takeout from our favorite Chinese restaurant. Jack is not a huge fan of Chinese food. "Beef chow mein, small portion please," is as far as he will go. I knew he wanted to do something to please me and to show that he is still capable of making decisions.

I called the order in and asked for the total of the bill so I could tell Jack and make it easier for him to pay. The total was going to be $15.15. When he came home he said he gave the woman a fifty, a ten and a five. She said that was too much and only needed fifteen cents. Lately he keeps pulling out fifties when we go to a restaurant. I think he figures that a fifty will cover the cost, whatever it is.

It reminds me of an anecdote that I read about a man with Alzheimer's who would do the same thing. Wherever he went, he would pull out fifty and one-hundred dollar bills, even for the smallest of purchases. His wife would cover for him and just say that she will pay because she has smaller bills.

Wednesday, October 19, 2005

UPS delivered the item Jack ordered on Sunday. He spent a lot of time in the bedroom. I was wondering if what was sent was the right thing.

As I began fixing dinner, he started to tell me that he has to return this thing with money by the thirtieth because **they** want it and if he doesn't **they** will cause trouble. I asked him if the item he received was what he wanted. He said, "Yes." Then there was no reason to return anything or send money. He had placed the order and used his credit card. The order was sent and his credit card was billed. The only time he needed to do anything was if he returned something.

He insisted that he had to send this because **they** want it. He even showed me the lower part of the statement which had a preprinted return label. Above it is a statement that says that no shipping will be charged for exchanges but $6.95 will be deducted from any refund amount for a returned item. This is what he was zeroing in on.

Tuesday, October 25, 2005

The local high school theatrical group is performing their fall play. Tricia and I decided to go to see it tonight. During the day I mentioned this to Jack several times so he would know we are going and where we would be. As we were leaving, I said that if the phone rang, he didn't need to answer it. The call would probably be for Tricia. Most of the evening calls are for her. Whoever called would leave a message.

When we returned home, Jack was upset. Some guy had called for me, gave his name and said he had just left the airport and was on his way here. I checked Caller ID but there weren't any unfamiliar names or numbers. Then I checked voicemail. There was one message from my brother saying, "Hi, this is Mudd, also known as your brother. I just left the airport and I'm on my way home." He hadn't called me in a while, hence the name Mudd. As usual, he had hoped to catch up with me and update our lives on the long drive to his home.

Tuesday, November 1, 2005

All Saints Day. Jack and I went to the 9 a.m. Mass at Holy Family Parish. The students from the new academy were in attendance. It was so good to see their fresh, happy faces. With few exceptions, most children start out the same. It is what happens to them and how they learn to deal with life that affects their development into adults.

I imagined Jack as the little boy with the innocent face of his First Communion photo. Then his blue eyes gazed serenely and happily from under the blond hair of his childhood. Now his face registered uncertainty, bewilderment, anxiety. Rarely is there a moment when peace floods his face and his features are relaxed. Usually his face relaxes only when he is tucked into bed. At last he does not have to think or remember. Sometimes during the early morning hours, I will lie quietly next to him just watching him sleep. It is the only time when he is truly peaceful. How much effort and energy every waking moment requires of him. Just the simple everyday activities demand an inordinate amount of concentration. Lately, he has been returning to bed each morning after breakfast. He looks exhausted and he is.

This afternoon we did a number of errands. We usually shop at a time when the stores are not busy. The less activity, the better it is for Jack. When we are together, and we are all the time now, Jack insists on paying the bills. It's fine with me. It takes longer but it is good for his self esteem and I won't do a thing to diminish that.

At one store, Jack needed $17.34. He pulled out his wallet and had a hard time figuring out what he needed. He pulled out two fifties, a twenty, then a hundred dollar bill. I encouraged him to use either a twenty or a fifty. Finally, he gave the teen-aged cashier a fifty. She said, "Boy, I wish I had such decisions to make!"

Sunday, November 13, 2005

Tear a month out of a calendar, cut it up into squares for each day and toss them in the air. That's how Jack perceives time. "Yesterday was Friday, so today is Tuesday, right?" So he has gone from "Tomorrow is garbage day, right?" to this.

Time of day is elusive as well. This is most noticeable relating to TV programming. Which also brings up the ability to use the remote. He has forgotten most channel numbers. And he knew them better than I. There is difficulty in punching in the correct numbers when he does know the combination. "**They** don't know how to make these things."

Elusiveness of time is what makes him get up at 3 a.m. on Sunday for 7:30 a.m. Mass. He gets dressed and eats "so I have the time I need." He used to sit in the family room until 7 a.m.

Recently, he will come back to the warm bed until I get up at 6:30. Sometimes he will get up earlier and wake me up, too, so I'm not late.

It has to be a most fearful thing to be somewhat aware that things are not right, but not know why or how. The intact parts of the brain know something is wrong, but the damaged parts prevent the brain from making an accurate assessment. The result must be like being in a maze. Every way you turn there is a dead end which creates more confusion and fear. There is an interior scream "I want out!" Fear escalates.

Thursday, November 17, 2005

Every year before Jack's birthday, Tricia and I always go to Woodfield Mall to shop. It's our day. Jack decided to come with, because he needed to shop, too. The three of us usually go the Monday after Thanksgiving to do Christmas shopping. Last year Jack forgot our meeting spot and panicked. This year, his grip on the date of any holiday is tenuous. So he thinks we are going shopping for Christmas.

This morning, he was up at 6:30 a.m. and had his coat on at 8 a.m. We told him the stores didn't open until 10 a.m. This is before Thanksgiving, not after. He said the parking lot would be full, if we went later. He was not going to join us. He would drive us there and drop us off because there wouldn't be any place to park.

Tricia and I finally convinced him to stay with us. We told him he would have his choice of spots, but he wasn't convinced. To ease his anxiety, we left home at 8:45 a.m. for the five-minute drive. When we drove into the covered parking area next to Nordstrom's, it was empty. He had his choice of every spot.

When we entered the mall, all the stores were closed. We put our coats into a locker and walked to the center of the mall, stopping at a kiosk for tea and a biscuit.

Jack insisted on going off on his own as he did every year. We decided to meet at The Cheesecake Factory for lunch. I prayed that he would remember where we were to meet and when. Before we left home, I had given him a slip of paper with my name and Tricia's on it and her cell phone number, just in case. He wouldn't be able to use it. But a store clerk or security person could call us. It was a good day. Jack remembered where to meet us for lunch.

At lunch he said that he had gone to Sears to look at the snow blowers. I know he is having difficulty trying to remember how to prep ours for winter. The instruction book no longer makes sense to him. Apparently he tried to ask a salesperson some questions. With his inability to verbalize what he wants to say, it was a loss. Every noun is becoming a *thing*.

After lunch, Jack wanted to go on his own again and we agreed to meet by the lockers at 3 p.m. Tricia and I crammed as much shopping as we could into two hours and were quite successful. As we walked along the upper level toward the bookstore around 2:30 p.m., I saw Jack just sitting on the lower level with his hands in his lap, waiting. He looked so alone, it is bringing tears to my eyes even as I write this.

I learned later that he had tried getting something "at that store back there but **they** don't know what **they** are doing." So he had nothing.

Friday, November 18, 2005

I mentioned to Jack that I earned cash back on my credit card. If I used my card to pay for the groceries, we could save two or three hundred dollars a year. He said, "Do it." Last year, he was adamant about paying the bill himself. Today, he made sure I had my card before we left home!

I am learning to be patient and bide my time. As an activity becomes more complicated and confusing, he will relinquish it. I cannot blame him for trying to hold on as long as he can. We all fear losing control. Last year, letting me pay for the groceries was not a smart economic move. In his mind, it was another small loss of control. While I saw it as good for us - he saw it as bad for him.

I've learned that there comes a time when the destruction in the brain makes the task overwhelming. Then there is an almost childlike relief in letting go. I am hopeful that this is what will happen with the gravest activity of all, driving. So far he has not lost any of his skills. When they begin to deteriorate, I pray that there will be a relinquishing of the keys without trauma.

Tuesday, November 22, 2005

Jack's seventy-sixth birthday. Tricia and I wished him a Happy Birthday at midnight. We asked him where he wanted to go for dinner on his birthday. He had no answer. I already had everything I needed to prepare a lobster dinner since the weather predictions for the day were less than desirable.

We have been so fortunate this fall. Until ten days ago, there were huge pink geraniums lining the walkway to the front door. Flowers in November in Illinois! Today was another beautiful fall day, despite the weather predictions. As storms sometimes do, this one zagged instead of zigged.

We decided to go to a seafood restaurant for dinner, instead. Jack accepted that it was his birthday. But all through dinner, he was concerned about when his sisters were coming and when the bags of leaves and yard waste needed to be put out.

"Are they coming for dinner today?"

"No. They are coming on Thanksgiving."

"They're coming tomorrow."

"No, Thursday. Tomorrow is garbage pickup day."

"I put it out tomorrow."

"We put it out tonight. It will be picked up tomorrow."

"Are they coming tomorrow?"
"They're coming on Thursday."
"When do I put the bags out again?"
"Tonight."
"Will they be here tonight?"
"They'll be here on Thursday, Thanksgiving Day."
And so it went.

Thursday, November 24, 2005

Thanksgiving Day. As we raised our glasses to toast the day, Jack said "Merry Christmas" and wasn't joking. His birthday, Thanksgiving, Christmas, New Years Day - they are all there somewhere. He just no longer knows where or in what order.

Yesterday he had his calendar on December and said, "This doesn't make any sense. There are squares here that are blank." November was in the wastebasket because he thought it was over with. I pulled it out of the basket and showed him how the 27th thru 30th of November filled in the squares in December. The understanding of the concept is totally gone.

Once again, my heart breaks because I think of all the years when he designed and directed those massive annual calendar programs for his company.

Monday, November 28, 2005

The sundowning aspect of Alzheimer's is occurring more frequently. In part, the shorter days as winter approaches may be contributing to it. The agitation level has ratcheted up a notch or two. The TV Guide no longer makes any sense. The remote is unfathomable if pushing the power button and the basic channels don't work. Except for looking at the sales ads, the newspaper is unreadable. The news channels so avidly watched for years are now becoming meaningless chatter. The activities that occupied fall and winter evenings for so many years are now a source of frustration.

Sundowning occurs in the moderate to late stages of dementia. It is characterized by cycles of increased confusion, anxiety, agitation and disorientation. Since these episodes occur most frequently at the end of the day or in the evening, they became known as sundowning. However, there isn't a true correlation between the episodes and the sun going down.

The causes are not fully understood, but appear to be more closely related to brain fatigue. A brain beset by dementia is always working hard to maintain functioning levels each day. In the morning when the brain has rested during sleep, it copes with the day's demands more easily. As the day progresses, the brain struggles to keep up. When it is overwhelmed, there is a melt down and an increased inability to distinguish that which is real from that which is not.

Tuesday, November 29, 2005

After eighteen years I have decided to fold the business to give one hundred percent of my attention to Jack. It has become more and more difficult to adhere to production schedules and still be there for him every time there is a problem. Earlier this year, I began to look through the sizeable inventory of fabrics, trims, ribbons and laces and use as much as I could to make doll costumes. These were placed in the stores at reasonable prices. This fall I have packed the spaces with finished inventory priced to sell. I hope to have very little left at year's end.

A few months ago, I toyed with the idea of just downsizing. Only keeping the most profitable stores and servicing those for another year. It is hard to let go completely. But the reality is that my time would still be divided. I must make a clean break. And so I am.

For the past few months I have been talking with Jack about my intentions. Today I gave the managers of the stores where I rent space notice that I would be vacating my spaces effective December 31st. After I had contacted them by phone, I followed up with written confirmation. I showed the letters to Jack and said I had finally bitten the bullet.

He said, "You mean we won't be going there, any more?"

"That's right."

"I didn't know that."

"That's what we've been talking about."

"You never told me. We won't be going to any of them?"

"We will go this week and a few times in December. But after Christmas, I'll pull everything out and it will be done."

Thursday, December 1, 2005

It is twenty-six years since Jack's mom died. There always was a special bond between Jack and his Mom. True, he was the youngest of her children and the only boy. But it was a mutual bond. It wasn't just a mom who doted on her son no matter what he did. Or a needy son who couldn't tear himself away from his mother's apron strings. It wasn't love hoping to gain something from the loving. The reciprocated love between mother and son was a profound love. Each knew both the other's strengths and weaknesses, yet loved unconditionally.

Throughout the years of our marriage when Jack's mom was alive, I was always in awe of that bond between the two and would never, ever do anything to compromise it.

This morning I asked Jack's mom to look after him in these trying times. I asked her to enfold her arms around her little boy and hold him tight. I asked her to intercede for me to God to give me the patience to show her son only love. And I asked her to greet her son with eternal joy when his pain and suffering are over. As if she wouldn't!

Friday, December 2, 2005

While Jack went to get a haircut, Tricia climbed into the crawl space and pulled out all the Christmas boxes. In past years it has been harder for him to crawl in and out, but he has refused all offers of help. Tricia was in and out like a flash, the wonders of young bones and muscles.

Saturday, December 3, 2005

Jack was quite tired today and slept a long time. Tricia and I brought up the boxes for the tree and began to set it up. When he awoke, he came into the living room and sat down and just watched us, something he never would have done before. And he never questioned how the boxes got out of the crawl space.

Tricia and I enjoyed putting up the tree. It was the first time in years when I could concentrate on the fun of it without thoughts of orders I had to fill and the costumes I still had to sew. More likely, being a Saturday, we wouldn't even be putting up the tree because I'd be doing a show.

In the evening I mentioned to Jack that the temperature was going down into the single digits Sunday night into Monday morning. We needed to switch the sump pump pipe so water wouldn't freeze in the ground. Wrong move. Should have waited until Sunday to mention it. Once I said something, he wasn't still. Fear again. He decided to get the pipe down from the rafters in the garage right away. He talked about getting up as soon as it was light. I reminded him that we had to go to Mass first.

Sunday, December 4, 2005

Jack didn't sleep but an hour. I was so tired, I slept until 6:30 a.m. Tricia was kept awake by his walking back and forth.

As soon as we returned from church, he set about changing the pipe. It had snowed an inch or so overnight which made the task harder. And it was cold. After the above ground pipe was connected and the sump pump ejected water into it without leaking, we had hot tea and toast. Then I tucked Jack into bed to warm up.

An hour later, he woke up asking where everyone was. I told him we were the only ones here. He and Tricia had been sleeping and I was doing paperwork. After a few minutes, he went back to bed and slept until mid afternoon. More and more frequently, he will fall asleep watching TV or take a nap. When he wakes up, he wants to know where everyone else is. Then he will shake his head in confusion.

Monday, December 5, 2005
We woke up at 7:30 a.m. today to go to Woodfield to do Christmas shopping. We left at 9 a.m., early enough to have a choice of parking spots in the covered lot near Nordstrom's. Shortly after we put our coats in a locker, Jack said his heel was bothering him and began favoring his left foot as he walked. We took an escalator to the upper level. He mis-stepped and almost fell. I was behind him and steadied him.

Tricia went off on her own. Jack and I stayed together. In one of the stores we used a down escalator. It, too, was a problem and I needed to steady Jack to prevent a fall. We purchased gifts for Tricia and Jack wanted to put them in the car before meeting her for lunch.

As we walked, he insisted on carrying the bag as always. He was still the gentleman. But it became more and more difficult for him to walk upright. He kept leaning to the right more and more to the point where it appeared that he could fall over at any second. I kept asking him to give me the bag, but he stubbornly refused.

When we neared the mall exit, he agreed to let me take the bag to the car while he waited. He was standing by the wall when I returned. Finally, he sat down to put his hanky in his shoe to buffer the pain of walking. When he took off his shoe, he found that the insert in the shoe had shifted and was causing the discomfort. As we made our way to the restaurant across the mall, he still held my hand and limped, but his walking was much better.

After lunch, I asked him if he still wanted to shop and he said, "Yes." He wanted to look for a coat for Tricia. Slowly we made our way around. Once again, we had to use an escalator to reach the upper level. Once again, he mis-stepped and had difficulty regaining his balance. If I had not been behind him, he would have fallen and taken a few people with him in the crowded mall. This one was quite scary.

We found a beautiful suede coat with faux leopard lining and trim and bought it. As we were walking down the aisle, Tricia came hurrying toward us. She had seen the perfect top to wear to a party she was attending and wanted to buy it. She selected the top and went into the fitting room with me to try it on while her dad waited.

Exiting the fitting room, I saw Jack holding onto a display. He did not look well and seemed to be in danger of falling. Since he had only had a hamburger at lunch, I thought that maybe his blood glucose level was dropping. I offered him hard candy. He refused it. He just wanted to leave.

Tricia still had to pay for her top. There were two cashiers at the station. One had a woman who was returning over $500 in merchandise. Every item had to be debited back to her account. The other cashier had a woman buying two packs of underwear whose prices couldn't be resolved. I thought we would never get out of the store.

As we left, Jack wasn't sure which way we were to walk. Again, he started leaning to the right as we walked. I had the coat in my left hand and a death grip on his left arm to steady him. I held my ground next to him and several people who wouldn't move over felt the impact of the bag with the coat. An eternity passed as we inched our way toward the elevator.

No more unstable escalators for him, especially not in this deteriorating condition. As soon as we stepped off the elevator, I had Jack sit on a stone wall. The sitting helped. Tricia hurried over to a shop to get a cup of regular pop, not diet. When she returned, Jack only drank about a quarter of the cup of pop.

After the brief rest we made it to the lockers. But the more Jack walked, the more he leaned to the right. However, once we got to the car which was parked near the entrance, he slid into the driver's seat and insisted on driving. And he was fine. He was alert and had no problems, whatsoever. Astounding! Ten minutes later, it was a relief to be home.

Jack took a blood glucose reading. Three hundred. So a low glucose level was not the problem. He only drank a quarter cup of the regular pop which wouldn't have raised his glucose level that much.

Recently, he mentioned that he had toppled off his desk chair (which has arms) while Tricia and I were out walking. Is this part of the dementia? A loss of cells in the area of the brain that controls balance? Would heel pain account for it? I can understand where heel pain would cause a limp and a tendency to favor that foot. But the leaning way over to the right is bizarre.

Now that we are at home, Jack is fine. I don't know how to explain it. I do know that I would not want to live it again.

Thursday, December 8, 2005

Last night I reminded Jack that we were going to Mass in the morning. So, naturally he was up at 5 a.m. I always know when he wakes up and gets out of bed. Then I turn over and try to get a little more rest. When I did get up at 6:30, Jack asked me "Where's dad? He told me that it didn't look like there would be a lot of snow. But he wasn't there when I looked around."

At lunch, he mentioned the episode. I asked him if he was dreaming. He said, "No, I was wide awake." A similar thing has happened a number of times over the past six months. Always he says he is not dreaming. But he doesn't understand it.

Wednesday, December 14, 2005

On Monday, Jack was up at 8 a.m. and didn't go to bed after breakfast. He was on a mission. He dressed and went off. When he returned around noon, he was upset. "**They** don't know what **they** are doing in those stores. **They're** stupid." Apparently he tried to Christmas shop. I know he couldn't verbalize what he was looking for and the stores do not have employees to give personal customer service. He was totally frustrated.

Yesterday, he put out with the garbage all the bags in the garage labeled for the Salvation Army with a big white card. Fortunately, he made a comment about having so much garbage. It gave me a clue as to what might have happened. We were able to retrieve the bags. Once again, "I never let him know what is going on." The big signs didn't mean a thing to him.

This morning, Jack had breakfast and went back to bed. I woke him about 12:30 p.m. and he ate a little lunch. Then, he lay down again and fell asleep. After dinner, he again slept until 10:30 p.m. I woke him up and he thought that it was morning. "Funny, it's still dark out."

Thursday, December 15, 2005

Forty years ago today was the Christmas party that started our personal relationship. That evening a group of coworkers had decided to go out for a drink after the in-house office dinner. One woman drove a group of people over to the lounge and so did I. Jack was among those in my car. By the time I parked the car and walked inside, there were only two seats left at the long table. Being the gentleman he has always been, Jack had waited and walked in with me. The seats were ours.

Another coworker of mine suggested that I try her favorite drink, a Manhattan. Thinking we were only going to have one drink and I was in the holiday spirit, I ordered one. The first taste made me realize how powerful a drink it is. There was a lively conversation going on at the far end of the table, but the noise level in the lounge made it impossible to join in.

Jack and I began our own conversation. It didn't take long for me to be intrigued by this man about whom I really knew nothing. As he spoke, I became aware of his intelligence, humor, perceptiveness, compassion. I became quite mesmerized by his conversation. I hardly noticed that two more rounds of drinks were ordered. As we were leaving the lounge, I was aware that we were holding hands. It was a perfect fit.

Jack was concerned that I was driving home and had another woman to drop off who lived further than I did. I was driving him and another fellow to the parking garage where he had his car. On the way he insisted we stop at a late night diner across from the parking garage for coffee. It is not one of my favorite beverages, but I sipped a little to ease his concern. I do remember driving down the South Lake Shore Drive feeling that the tires were not touching the pavement.

The date does not mean anything to Jack anymore. He may not know the why of an occasion, but he relishes the special meals. I revel in his enjoyment and feel the need to celebrate all occasions together, however we can, whenever we can, while we still can.

What would I have thought forty years ago had I known the future? It was all joy the next day when Jack stopped by my desk and asked me to go to lunch with him. Would knowing the future have made a difference in my answer? No. Because the night before I saw a facet of this man I didn't know existed and it captured my heart.

I just keep redoubling my prayers to the Lord that He give me patience. I am truly learning how to take one day at a time. It really is all I can handle. And He has not failed me. I feel blessed that much of the knowledge I acquired while doing research on developmental disabilities and minimal brain dysfunction when our daughter was in special ed classes so many years ago is again being put to good use. So much of it can be translated and reversed in comprehending how the mind of an Alzheimer's victim works - or doesn't.

Monday, December 19, 2005

Keeping another yearly tradition, Tricia and I spent the weekend baking hundreds of cookies of all sizes and flavors and description. It is a marathon event that fills the kitchen and the house with warmth and delicious aromas. For twenty years our neighbors and relatives have eagerly awaited the results of this marathon. Each year a few more recipients are added to the list and so the number of pans of cookies continues to grow.

Tonight Tricia went with a friend to see a Christmas play. Her dad was solicitous about whether she had enough money. He gave her fifty dollars and wanted to know if she needed more. Tricia was amazed because her dad had never given her that much spending money. This was a win-win situation. She was delighted to have the extra money. Her dad was happy that he was able to do what dads do.

Tuesday, December 20, 2005

For a few days, Jack has been quite frustrated because his attempts to shop for Christmas gifts have ended in failure. He has always spent much time and effort in shopping for thoughtful gifts. Not being able to do so this year was a monumental change in his abilities.

Every year he would worry that there wouldn't be enough wrapping paper for all the gifts. "I need a big roll. I have two BIG boxes to wrap." Every year I would assure him that there was plenty of paper and every year he would doubt that there would be. In itself the exchange of conversation became a yearly tradition.

When Jack wrapped a gift, the paper would be cut to the exact measurement for each different sized box. The ribbons and bows were attached just so. Absolute perfection, the artist at work.

Last night Jack said he wanted to go shopping with me this morning to get something new like a coat. He's big on coats. I could do nicely with the two I have which he gave me two years ago. (That year he outdid himself in giving. It was almost like his last hurrah. I sometimes wonder if he did it because he sensed that things were not right and he was going to do what he could while he could. I will never know.)

Jack was upbeat, a rarity these days. "We'll go to Marshall Fields. You can look at all the coats and you could use new boots. And we can get your favorite mints."

We were up early and at Woodfield mall by 8 a.m. For as eager as he was to do this last evening, today it cost him a lot personally. Again he had great difficulty walking and he was unsteady but he was also determined. I found a beautiful black cashmere and merino wool coat that had excellent tailoring and design at a good price. Jack was happy.

But his face looked drained. All the enthusiasm to look for boots and candy and other items was forgotten. Time to go home. He was shaky stepping onto the escalator going up. I stepped on behind him to steady him, if necessary. How different from all the years when this gentleman would always let a lady, especially his wife, precede him.

Jack was pleased that he had been able to gift me. He loves me and still wants to show that love. But at what price!

These last few words just flowed from the pen as fast as the tears they have unleashed from my eyes. He has always given every bit of himself to others. Whatever needed doing, he has done it without heed of the cost to himself. His determination and perseverance were boundless.

We were home by 9 a.m.

Saturday, December 24, 2005

Christmas Eve. The house is sparkling, the presents are wrapped, the baking is done and delivered to the neighbors. No longer having to tend to endless production for the stores has its advantages.

Jack was surprised when I served his favorite dinner, even though I kept reminding him all day that it was Christmas Eve. He did enjoy it immensely. There is so little he can truly enjoy, it gives me great satisfaction just to see his pleasure. After dinner, he asked if this was the night he should put the garbage out. Sigh!

Around 11 p.m., I called LaVerne to see if she was home safely. For many years she has gone to a friend's house for Christmas Eve. She intended to go this year. As usual, Lee is out of town visiting her daughter. This time before she left, she took LaVerne on a dry run of the route she needed to drive. LaVerne had driven it many, many times before and Lee said she'd be fine. I was not so sure.

LaVerne said she had gotten lost going and coming. But guardian angels had helped her out. She said she stopped at a restaurant on the way there. The manager said he didn't know where she wanted to go. As she stood outside, a man approached and said he would take her there. She followed him to her friend's. Regarding the return, she made a cryptic comment. "The woman said her son would help as soon as he finished his ham sandwich." ???

I reminded her that she was coming here tomorrow, Christmas Day. I had a specific cab driver who would pick her up. He knows how to get here. She will stay overnight so she should pack her bag.

Sunday, December 25, 2005

Christmas Day. Awoke at 6:30 a.m. It was sleeting outside. The driveway and roads were slick. Fortunately, Jack said he didn't want to drive in such weather and went back to bed. I thanked God that I did not have to talk him out of driving. I did not want to miss Mass on Christmas Day of all days, but we were doing our best.

The storm passed. By 10 a.m. the streets were clear. I couldn't get Jack up and ready for the 11 o'clock Mass. He no longer moves quickly. We had breakfast and then settled in the living room by the tree to open our gifts. Tricia was ecstatic with her camera phone and the new suede coat. Jack was happy with the fleece lined jacket shirts we gave him among other things.

But he was upset that he had not done more. In the midst of opening a gift, he got up and left the room. When he returned he gave Tricia a plain envelope with money in it. I know he had just put it together in the bedroom. How different from years past when he would have purchased a thoughtful card and done this well in advance.

At the end of our gift giving, he disappeared again. When he returned, he had the brown delivery box from the catalog company. Inside was the item he had had so much trouble ordering in October. It is a beautiful faux fur jacket!

At noon, I called LaVerne to remind her that the cab would pick her up at 2 p.m. I asked her if she had her overnight bag ready. "Am I staying overnight? I didn't know I was." That put her into a tizzy. Told her I was hanging up so she could put her nightgown and makeup and medicine in her bag.

At 2:45 p.m., the cab driver drove up with LaVerne. Nice guy. Handled the situation well. No repeat of last year.

LaVerne wasn't in the house ten minutes when I could hear her voice and Jack's escalating in the living room. She was telling Jack her tale about Lee wanting to move to where her daughter lives. She wants LaVerne to go with. Because Jack has not heard this story five thousand times, he was saying that his sister had a right to live where her daughter was if that's what she wants. LaVerne was adamant that her sister couldn't leave her. I couldn't tell Jack in front of LaVerne that she has told me this story two or three times every time we talk on the phone. No one has any intention of moving anywhere. Ignore it!

Monday, December 26, 2005

Fourteen of my family members came for dinner and our holiday get together. They arrived at 1 p.m. and left at 5 p.m. Tomorrow is a work day. I am so indebted to them for making the long trek up here from the south suburbs and Indiana. It was a sacrifice to come so far for such a short time. It did my heart so much good to see them.

The dinner was stressful for Jack. LaVerne kept asking him who the different relatives were. He has a time of it remembering himself. Especially since we haven't seen them in a while. And she won't let up because when you tell her, she forgets and asks again and again and again. It aggravates Jack because then he has to try and remember again and again and again.

Tuesday, December 27, 2005

Another bittersweet day. I pulled the last of the doll clothes inventory out of the stores. It is the end of a long run of eighteen years, a good one at that. It is also a big relief. For now there is nothing to divert my attention from Jack and our life together.

Saturday, December 31, 2005

This has been a year of great losses for Jack. He no longer knows how old he is. In March, he lost the meaning of all the columns on his diabetic chart. After much stress and trauma, he relinquished the checkbook and writing of checks and seemed relieved to do it. He could no longer remember how to service the lawnmower. He finally agreed to my help in taking his blood glucose readings and insulin injections. He is forgetting how to work the TV remote. He can no longer shop on his own because he is unable to communicate what he wants. He is gradually losing knowledge of when to go to church and why. Last year, he signed Tricia's cards 'From Your Father'. This year he never thought to buy cards. The days of the week are a total fog and months are missing.

◊◊◊◊◊◊◊◊◊◊

CHAPTER EIGHT

Sunday, January 1, 2006
    This morning I prayed the prayer of acceptance, knowing full well that it will be a year with a lot of pain and grief. There will be joy to be treasured. The disease will encroach inexorably. What will be lost next is unknown.
    Since I no longer have production schedules, I pray I will have more patience. I hope to use reading - even a few novels which I haven't read in years - as my escape when stress builds. It worked when I was a child, taking me out of my surroundings for a time. Enough to reinforce hope and build up strength to face the present.
    Sometimes, at least for a moment, I still can't believe that this is occurring. With Jack being diabetic, I always thought we would be facing a totally physical problem together. Never did I ever think of Alzheimer's.

Wednesday, January 4, 2006
    We were watching the news coverage of a mining disaster in West Virginia. A commercial aired showing a maple tree with a chute for sap being inserted into its bark. At first, sap came trickling out of the tree down the chute, then squares of cereal. The ad inference being that eating the cereal was like eating maple syrup itself.
    Jack looked at it and said, "**They** can't do that, can **they**?"
    The ubiquitous **they**. No matter what happens, **they** are the culprits. It could be the weather, arthritis pain, or a problem. No matter what it is he cannot understand, **they** are the cause.
    He is definitely losing his grip on the reality of what he sees on TV, whether it is happening now or it is from the past.

Tuesday, January 10, 2006

Jack had his checkup with the endocrinologist. Last time, he was aggravated because the doctor came out to speak with me. (Once again, I am relegated to the waiting room.) Jack told the doctor that he did not want him to do that. He could take care of things. As we were waiting for paperwork to be completed, the doctor sauntered by, greeted me, and casually mentioned that he had given Jack a new prescription for high blood pressure. Then he continued on. But he had done what he intended to do - let me know what was going on. I appreciated his thoughtfulness.

On the way home, Jack said that the doctor was concerned about his blood pressure. He had told the doctor that it was like that when he was in Korea and the medic next to him told him it was okay and not to worry.

Recently, any time a question arises about blood glucose or blood pressure readings, he maintains it's been like that since he was in Korea (54 years ago). Apparently that is where he is in his mind at the present time.

Thursday, January 12, 2006

It's forty years since Jack proposed to me. I thought about mentioning it at breakfast, then decided against it. He was too focused on what **they** were doing with the winter weather. Two different men, the one sitting at table with me today and the one who proposed forty years ago.

The night Jack proposed, I knew I would rather spend six months with him, than a lifetime with someone else. That's what my heart knew. My mind cautioned me. We had only dated three weeks. I could be setting myself up for heartbreak. I followed my heart that night and never regretted it.

Jack has never broken my heart. Until now. It is breaking not because of any action of his, but because of that which he is powerless to control, this disease.

THEY LIVED AT OUR HOUSE

Monday, January 16, 2006

Jack often goes back to bed after breakfast. He looks so worn out. His face is drawn and he shuffles along on those hereditarily thin legs. Tucking him in under the comforter and the lap robe Tricia gave him is like tucking in a little boy totally worn out by his day and eager for blissful slumber.

Oftentimes, he will awaken suddenly, walk out of the bedroom and ask where everyone went or where we have to go. "Weren't my sisters here?" or "Don't we have to go to Mass?" or "Where are we supposed to go?"

After I reassure him that we are the only three here and there is no where we need to be, he'll shuffle back to bed.

Today, he was perplexed. After late morning tea and toast, he was alert, but said,

"She keeps asking me to visit. I don't see how I can do that."

"Who keeps asking you to visit?"

"She's asked me several times, but I don't see how I can do that."

I asked again, "Who?"

"Mother. But I don't know how I can do that. They're not there anymore. I don't understand it."

"Where is there?"

"You know, where they used to be, you know, there."

"Not here?"

"No. There where they used to be, where everything was, where they lived."

"Where you grew up?"

"Yes, that's it. But I don't understand how I am going to do that. There must be other people living there now."

His face showed the perplexity he felt and the confusion. Never once did he say, and the thought did not occur to him, that it was impossible because his parents had died over twenty years ago.

When I sought to ease his mind by calling the situation a dream, he rejected it. I didn't know what I was talking about. This was not a dream. It was real. But he didn't understand it. Sometimes during these occurrences, I imagine tiny cells of his brain suddenly going dark or flaking off - one here, one there. The remaining ones are trying to do their best to bridge the gaps. Like pixels on a computer or TV screen that start to burn out, one here, one there. At first, it isn't too noticeable. The picture is still easy to absorb and understand. But as more and more go black with ever increasing randomness, the picture is more indecipherable, the message more unreadable.

Sunday, January 29, 2006
By the grace of God, the week before this last one was easy. Just the usual glitches, no cataclysmic happenings. God knew how much time I would spend on the phone with LaVerne. Lee left town for a week on the previous Saturday.

Last Sunday, before I had a chance to call her, LaVerne was on the phone.

"When is my sister coming back?"

"Saturday."

"She told me to call her neighbor because he's sick and find out how he is. But I don't have his number. I called a number I had but they told me it was disconnected."

"LaVerne, the neighbor is fine now. You told me this story at Christmastime."

"Well, I know she told me. I wouldn't make this up. That's the trouble with her, she leaves the middles out of everything. When did you say she was coming back?"

"Saturday."

"Well, she certainly has it easy. She doesn't have a care in the world. When is she coming back?"

"Saturday."

As usual this was followed by the often told stories about her neighbors and their leaves and branches being dumped into her yard and the grown son saying his father told him not to talk to her, etc. etc.

On Monday, we had a repeat of the same conversation in the morning about 11 a.m.

On Tuesday, she called around 2 p.m. She told me she had a plumber out. Her kitchen sink wouldn't work. He came out and fixed it. It cost three hundred dollars. But everything is okay. He charged too much. He told her to call him if she needs more work. He would give her a better price.

I tried to find out exactly what was wrong, but never got a straight answer. Who was the guy? What was his name? What did he do? Where was the receipt?

She was more interested in when Lee was coming back. We went through this same dialogue and stories as we did on Sunday and Monday.

Wednesday's phone call was a long repeat of Tuesday's.

On Thursday, she called me at 9 a.m.

"When is she coming back?"

"Saturday. How are you doing?"

"Terrible, I don't have any hot water."

"What do you mean you don't have any hot water?"

"I don't have any hot water."

"In the kitchen?"

"No! Everywhere. I have to boil it, if I need hot water."

"When did this happen?"

"It's been like this ever since that jerk was here. I should have called the police. That's what you get for taking a name out of a magazine."

"Did you get it from the newspaper or phone book?"

"I don't remember where I got it from."

"What was his name?"

"He wouldn't give me his name."

"His name should be on the receipt or in your checkbook."
"I didn't pay him by check. I gave him cash."
"Why?"
"He said it would be thirty dollars more if I paid by check."
"I'm surprised that you had that much cash. You never have that much cash."
"I wish I didn't. I should have called the police. Everything happens to me..."
I interrupted. "Is there water available in all the sinks and for flushing the toilet?"
She assured me there was. Just no hot water. Then she said, "Well, I'm not going to worry about it. I called my friend and we're going to lunch at one o'clock and to a movie. She said she could help me. But I don't want too many people involved."
Then we went through the litany of stories about the neighbors. Finally, I interrupted her again and asked if she were dressed. She said 'no'. I suggested that it would be a good thing to dress so she would be ready when her friend came.
"I don't even remember what time she is coming."
"You told me one o'clock."
Her tone throughout the latter part of the conversation was light because she was going out with someone.
I called her later in the day to see how lunch had gone. She was pleased because her friend's husband had joined them.
"He's such a good looking man. We went to a very nice restaurant. They only go to the best places. He had to leave and return to work but we sat and talked."
Eventually the conversation turned to the lack of water. She said,
"I don't want to tell anyone else. I'll wait until she comes back and gives me the name of that plumber. He was here a while back and he told me the water wasn't hot enough and I should get it replaced. But you never know if they are telling you the truth or trying to make money."

"What did he say needed replacing? The water heater?"

"I guess so. You just can't trust them and they talk so fast I can't remember everything they say. When did you say she was coming back?"

"Saturday, the day after tomorrow."

The remainder of the conversation dealt with paperwork that was overwhelming to her, the banks not knowing what they were doing (sounds familiar) and the stories about the neighbors.

On Friday, I called. LaVerne was upset.

"Everything is against me. I made this phone call and the woman said they didn't take care of that and transferred me and the next thing I knew I was talking to someone in Texas. Can you imagine! I'll probably have to pay for it. That horrible bank. No bills. No receipts. When is she coming back?"

"Late tomorrow."

"Thank God. I have a bunch of stuff for her. Ever since she left, there's been no hot water. It couldn't be the worst time. She's got it made. I've got sh..... I hate this time of year. All the paperwork and the taxes. Somebody called but I can't remember why. They transferred me to Texas. Betcha I'll have to pay fifty dollars for that bill."

After hearing all the stories about the leaves and the neighbors, I did some questioning. I am reasonably sure that the phone call all the way to Texas was about her medication which she orders by mail.

On Saturday, LaVerne called about 1:30 p.m.

"When is she coming home?"

"Late today. Lee might be delayed because of the rainy weather. She has a stopover in St. Louis."

"I don't have any heat."

"When did this happen?"

"Today."

"Look at the thermostat. Is it on 'ON'?"

"Wait a minute." She put the phone down. "It's 99."

THEY LIVED AT OUR HOUSE

"Is it on 'Heat'?
"Let me check." Phone down. "It's 99."
"What is the temperature?"
"Hold on." Phone down. "It's 99."
"It can't be 99. You'd be roasting in the house."
"I wish my husband was here. He would always say 'I'll take care of it. Go out and have a good time.' Why did he have to die? What is it about widows that God likes so much that He makes so many of them? How I wish I could die in my sleep. Then you'd have to do all the paperwork."
LaVerne called at 12:30 p.m. today (Sunday).
"That sister of mine. I went to church and my friend invited me for brunch. I said 'no' because my sister was waiting for me. When I got home she was there screaming at me because I was late and her friends were waiting. She knows my Mass is later than hers. She said the hot water heater was turned off and I should call the guy next door. Then she walked out. If I had known that I could have gone to brunch. I can't call the guy next door. He's an accountant. His wife always calls people to get things done."
"I'm sure he knows how to start the pilot on a water heater. What about the heat?"
"It's fine."
"Are you getting heat in the registers?"
"Everything's okay. She said it was off. That guy said he was going to turn the hot water off when he fixed the plumbing so it wouldn't be wasted."
"You never told me that on Tuesday."
"I don't remember. I haven't had heat or hot water since he was here."
"You had heat. You called yesterday to say that it wasn't working. You told me on Thursday that the hot water wasn't working since the plumber was there on Tuesday. But the heat is on now, it's coming through the registers?"

"Yes. If I'd known that I could have gone to brunch with my friend. But that's all my sister has on her mind is that her girlfriends are waiting for her."

"LaVerne, if you lived in a small place, you wouldn't have to worry. You could have closed the door and gone to brunch with your friend."

"You say that because you're young. I don't want to move and end up hating my husband for making me move."

"How could you hate him? If something happens to Jack, I won't stay here forever. I feel blessed that we've had this lovely house for all these years but I won't hold on to it forever. I'll find a place that's smaller and requires less maintenance. I'll take the happy memories with me. But I certainly wouldn't blame Jack! Most people downsize as they get older to avoid all the maintenance."

Then she said for the thousandth time, "What is it that God likes about widows? There are so many of them. He takes all the men."

In total frustration, and tongue-in-cheek, I replied, "God is portrayed as a Man, isn't He? Well, widows can spend all their time praising him and praying to Him when they don't have a husband to look after! Like any Man, He wants their undivided attention."

The conversation deteriorated from there. It was a rehash of the entire week over and over.

More than likely, LaVerne was fiddling with the thermostat again hoping to save money. She needs to be someplace where if there is a problem, someone is on hand to check it out. As her memory worsens, she will have more problems because she is always fiddling with things. As it is, she's had problems with her car not starting because she fiddles with the light switch which leaves the lights on and drains the battery. She panics when the washing machine won't fill because in her penny pinching ways she turns the water volume down too low.

THEY LIVED AT OUR HOUSE

Wednesday, February 1, 2006
　　LaVerne called to tell me her microwave died and now she has a new one. "I'm so lucky to have a sister who knows what to do and where to go." She was as mellow as could be.
　　What a difference three days have made. After a week of storm clouds and negativity, all is sunshine and roses with her.

Thursday, February 2, 2006
　　But one knows that with Alzheimer's the sunshine never lasts long enough. LaVerne called early in the morning.
　　"I don't have any water."
　　"In the kitchen?"
　　"Yes."
　　"Is the water running in the bathroom?"
　　"Yes."
　　"Call the plumber and let him know. Then call me back."
　　After a few minutes, the phone rang.
　　"I don't have any water in the bathroom, either."
　　"Maybe the city shut the water off."
　　"I remember somebody saying that...."
　　"Call the city and find out what's going on. Call me back."
　　After another few minutes, LaVerne called back.
　　"I called. They said there's a water main break outside my house. There are trucks all over. One is in my driveway. I don't want him there. I'm going to get dressed and tell him to move his truck. They'll ruin the driveway."
　　"Did you call the plumber?"
　　"I've got to tell that guy off. I don't want him on the driveway."
　　"Did you call the plumber?"
　　"That guy shouldn't be on my driveway."
　　"Did you call the plumber?!?"
　　"Yes. He's coming out."

"Well you'd better call him back. There's nothing wrong in the house. You'll have to pay a service call fee if he comes out. Call him."

A few minutes go by and the phone rings for the fourth time.

"I keep calling. I can't get the plumber. I've got to tell that man."

"They're fixing your water main. Don't be nasty. I'll see if I can get through to the plumber."

Called the plumber and was told that the appointment had been canceled. LaVerne couldn't remember a few minutes later because she was focused on the truck in her driveway.

Later in the day, the phone rang again.

"My TV isn't working!"

Lee said she would go by and see what was wrong with the TV. She called me later. When she walked into LaVerne's house, she asked her what was wrong with the TV.

LaVerne replied, "Who said anything was wrong with the TV?"

It was the new microwave. She did not remember that she had to press the stop button twice to get the time back on.

Meanwhile, back at the ranch, Jack decided that he was going to the bank with his pension check. I asked him if he had a deposit slip. He looked blank. Asked him if he wanted me to write one out. What did he want to do with the check? Deposit all of it? Take all in cash? Or take some cash and deposit the rest? It was too much for his mind to comprehend and we went over and over it for twenty minutes.

He kept saying he wanted to put this amount in (pointing to the written amount) and take this out (pointing to the numeric amount). I wrote out sample deposit slips but he rejected them. I could do no more and let him leave. Maybe he could tell the bank teller what he wanted and she could fill out a slip. It was a long shot but I was exhausted from going round and round.

Jack came home without any transaction being made. "**They** don't know what **they're** doing. Finally he said he wanted to 'put it all in.' I wrote out a deposit slip. He said he was taking it to the main bank because "at this other one **they** don't know what **they're** doing." I asked if he wanted me to come with. I waited in the car while he went in and had no problem depositing the check.

A good synonym for caregiver is tightrope walker. A caregiver must assume so many of the tasks that the person with dementia is no longer capable of handling independently. But every step must be taken with utmost care. One too many steps at the wrong time and destruction looms. The caregiver must learn how to do something for the other person without letting that person know that it is you and not they who are doing it.

Friday, February 3, 2006
Awoke at 4:30 a.m. Jack said, "This isn't right."
"What isn't right?"
"These numbers," pointing to the digital clock on the bedside table. "They keep going up."
"They are supposed to. It's a clock." I could tell that the idea it was a clock was not registering. I felt Jack's skin. It was warm and dry so it wasn't a hypoglycemic reaction. Just to be on the safe side, I suggested he take a glucose reading. It was good.

We lay down again and every minute, Jack would turn and say, "41." "42." "43."
"Jack, stop looking at the clock."
"44."
"Jack, go to sleep."
"45. It keeps going up."
"It's supposed to. It's a clock."
"46. Something's not right."
"It will keep on going up until it reaches 59."

"47."
"Jack, stop looking at the clock. Turn over on your back."
"48."
"Jack, turn over on your right side." (Away from the clock)
"49."
"50."
"51."
"Jack, if you don't stop announcing the number, I'm going to announce you into oblivion."
"52."
"53."
"54."
Sigh. He finally fell asleep at 6 a.m.

Friday, February 10, 2006

About 2 a.m., static electricity set off the doorbell in the foyer. The doorbell can be programmed to play one of 25 different tunes when the bell is pressed. Usually when lightning or static electricity set it off, it will play a tune and that is that. Tonight we awoke and thought we died and had gone to heaven. The notes were going up and down the scale in waves of sound like a harp. There was no stopping it by changing the levers for the tune or pressing the doorbell. It quit playing when the connection in the basement was touched. Then it wouldn't work at all. Once all was quiet, it was back to bed.

Jack did not sleep at all. Fixing the doorbell was on his mind. He was fully dressed at 7 a.m. After breakfast, he went downstairs and started adjusting the screw. I heard little ticking sounds in the doorbell when the connection was made. The bell was back in business. Thankfully, this was one of the things that Jack remembered how to do without any problem. One can only stand in awe of the human mind. What a marvel it is when it is fully functional. And how perplexing it is when it is not.

Sunday, February 12, 2006

The night sprite was flitting about at 5 a.m. this morning. He was ready to awaken Tricia when she called out, "Daddy, it's only 5. We don't get up until 6:30." She has really shown so much patience with her dad. I know she does not understand why he is acting this way and it is confusing for her. This is her dad. Yet, when asked to accept whatever happens, she does. She is beautiful in her patience.

After church, we were sitting sipping cups of hot tea. Jack said, "It doesn't look good. I don't want to go and get the short ones. I need the long ones. If you go, you will get the wrong thing. You'll only get two and it won't be worth it."

How hard it is to understand what he is trying to say at times. Since the dementia began, he has steadily lost his communication skills. First, proper names of famous people and places and things. Then, common nouns began to disappear into thin air or were used interchangeably causing much confusion. Pronouns, especially **they**, have held their own. It has become more difficult to verbalize what he wants to say. I know the thought is there in his mind. The problem is translating it into vocabulary. And now even the timbre of his voice is decreasing. He has begun to speak much more softly.

This has created another problem. Jack has always been a quiet man. But the tone of his voice was always understandable. With the decline in volume, it has become necessary at times to ask him to repeat what he said. Since it was so difficult to get it out in the first place, it is a source of agitation for him.

Once again, your heart breaks. You watch helplessly as he becomes more and more isolated from everyone and everything.

Sunday, February 19, 2006

Time has lost its meaning totally. Jack was up at 1:30 a.m., dressed and sitting in the family room all ready for 7:30 a.m.

Mass. At 5:30 a.m., he was in the bedroom telling me it was time to get dressed or we would be late. By the time Tricia and I were ready as usual at 7 a.m., he was upset. **They** are always changing things. **They** should leave things alone. Why are **they** changing the Mass times?

His aggravation was still there when we were leaving. I had to remind him that he had shifted the car into Drive before he put his foot on the gas to back out of the garage. We could have had a drive-thru dining room. This is the first time that his aggravation has affected his driving skills. That is a concern.

On the way to church, I prayed that God will use His almighty power to resolve the driving, if it becomes an issue. How do you take away the keys? It is one of the most sensitive issues to be dealt with when a person should no longer be driving because of physical or mental changes. I am asking God to do as He sees fit. It is all in His hands.

I reminded myself that He resolved the checkbook and budget issues and my need to know how much insulin Jack was taking and when. And He did it all in placid ways. This problem, too, I turn over to Him to resolve without accident or tragedy occurring.

Wednesday, February 22, 2006

The dryer gave up the ghost. In December the latch broke and fell into the door. Tricia and I have been pushing the step stool with heavy detergent bottles on it against the door to keep it tightly shut so the dryer would work. Now it will not heat up.

Thank heaven for the internet. Before I mentioned to Jack that we needed a new dryer, I went online. I was able to look at all the different models, compare features and decide on two or three that might work. Then we went to Sears. It was a pleasant experience because there weren't too many choices or too much information to deal with.

Even restaurants are becoming a problem. There are too many choices on the menu. Jack has resorted to ordering breakfast wherever we go. But even that is now problematic. After placing an order for the dryer, we stopped for lunch. Jack was concerned because the menu stated "Two eggs with your choice of 3 strips of bacon, 3 sausage links or 3 patties." He thought that he would get all of that and he only wanted bacon. I reassured him that if he ordered eggs with bacon, that is all he would get. He still thought he was going to get the wrong thing. He was uneasy until the waitress brought his plate exactly as he had ordered it.

For dinner we had ham sandwiches and potato salad. I saw Jack pick up a big spoonful of potato salad from the bowl. When I looked at his plate, there was none on it. Then I noticed that he had put the potato salad between the ham and cheese in his sandwich. Maybe he's invented a new deli creation.

In the evening, we were watching a channel on TV that had a program featuring animals and their crazy antics. In some of the segments the animals were hilarious and Jack was laughing heartily. Tricia leaned over and whispered to me, "Now that's the Daddy I remember."

Wednesday, March 1, 2006
Pension check cashing time again. Jack put on his coat and hat and said he was going to the bank. I asked if he wanted a deposit slip. Another go around, same as last month. That's not the way he has been doing it. He's been doing this for years. He's not going to that mickey mouse branch. He's going to the one where **they** knew what **they** were doing last time. I said nothing and let him go.

Fifteen minutes later, I answered the phone.
"Hello, this is the senior personal banker at Harris Bank. Your husband John is here with his pension check, which I

assume he wants to deposit. Can you please tell me if this is correct?'

"As far as I know, yes."

"I noticed on your records that a similar deposit was made last month."

"That's correct."

"Okay, we'll take care of it for him."

"Thank you. I appreciate your diplomacy in handling this."

"Let me give you my personal number in case you ever need assistance with banking problems."

He gave me the number and I thanked him again. I presumed that Jack did not know that he called me. It was an intelligent and compassionate way of dealing with the situation.

When Jack came home, he was upset. "The last time I was there, I had no problem. (Because you had a deposit slip.) There was a young girl and she knew what to do.

"This time I got this old woman and she didn't know what she was doing. And she called another old woman. I kept telling her this goes to me and this has to go there and then it has to go there and then they send it back to me. But she wouldn't listen. Then another woman came over and she was talking to some guy. **They** don't know what **they** are doing. **They** gave me this paper but it's not right. **They** are taking money. I don't trust them. It should go to California or somewhere. It's all screwed up." And so it went for ten minutes.

As he began to calm down, I asked Jack if he had the transaction receipt.

"Yes, but it's not right. **They** are taking money for college. We're not going to college. I don't trust that bank. I need to call that place and let them know what **they** are doing."

"What place?" I wasn't sure what he was talking about.

"That place. You know, that place where I used to work."

"They wouldn't know about this. It's handled for them by another bank."

THEY LIVED AT OUR HOUSE

Finally, he gave me the transaction receipt. Everything was okay. On the bottom was a line that read "Get Help for College with a Harris Home Equity." That's what bothered Jack.

"Jack, it's just an advertisement to drum up business. I showed him past transaction receipts with similar ads on them. But I could not dissuade him from the thought that something was wrong. He was going to let his past employer know that something wasn't right.

He tried looking for the phone number in the telephone directory, but couldn't find it. Another skill that is lost. Then he started going through his files. This is one of the times when it is prudent not to be helpful. Somewhere there is an unsuspecting employee who doesn't need any unsolicited aggravation.

By the end of the afternoon, Jack had calmed down. He couldn't find the number. I just kept repeating, "Everything is okay. The money is in the account. It's okay."

Thursday, March 2, 2006

In the course of looking for the phone number yesterday, Jack found the catalyst for today's problem. It came in the form of a letter from Ford regarding the Mercury. All morning and again after lunch, Jack was out in the garage. He finally came in totally aggravated. When I asked him what was wrong, he said,

"**They** don't know what **they** are talking about. I've been on the floor looking under the car and there is no place to put those things."

"What things?"

"I'll show you." He handed me a sheet showing how to jack up the car to change a flat tire using the spare.

"Jack, the tires are fine. Why would you want to do that?"

"This came in the mail yesterday. Those buzzards want you to call, but **they** might not be able to do it right away. I'll go in but if **they** can't do it right away, the heck with them."

The packet of information contained a letter explaining that there could be problems jacking up the car using the current directions. The packet also contained a new instruction sheet for the owner's manual; a new sticker to replace the current one located under the tire in the trunk, and instructions on replacing the sticker yourself. The letter said the car owner could take the car to the dealership to have it done which might require a wait. It was easy to do and many people could do it themselves.

The letter was dated September 2000. To Jack, it might as well have been yesterday. When I mentioned the date to him, it made no difference. Also mentioned that the new sticker was supposed to go under the spare tire, not under the car.

How it wounds the heart to know that he cannot fully comprehend what he reads. His world is getting smaller and smaller as abilities are being destroyed. Where will it end?

Saturday, March 4, 2006

Two years ago, when Alzheimer's seemed to be the logical answer to what was afflicting Jack, I felt strong. I can handle this. I am not a stranger to deficiencies in the brain. I felt calm and fully equipped to be patient, learn all I could, accommodate, adapt, innovate. Recently, my body is reintroducing me to the symptoms I lived with in the last stressful years before Jack's dad died. So many headaches, all sorts of aches and pains, and the constant feeling of being on edge. Anything can trigger an episode. One is never relaxed, waiting for the other shoe to drop.

Tricia becomes upset because she equates these episodes with the angry conversations that are had by couples whose marriages are falling apart. Many times she has been reassured that that is not happening. This is the result of her dad's disease.

This is the Catch 22 of the situation. As Alzheimer's destroys more and more pieces of Jack's brain, his intelligence has a more difficult time trying to make sense of what is going on each day. So he becomes frustrated at the **"they"** creating the confusion.

No matter how many times I tell Tricia that her dad cannot control what he says or does because of the disease, she gets upset. Jack's failing mind no longer allows him to remember her limitations. These limitations make it very difficult for her to remember that her dad's mind is failing him.

It is hard being in the middle.

Thursday, March 9, 2006

LaVerne and Lee came for dinner today. There is a decided decline in LaVerne since I saw her at Christmas. As her memory of events fails, she tries to fill in the gaps with information she has heard. She started talking about the house she gave to her parents and Lee reminded that she never did any such thing. She kept repeating this and each time she was reminded. On the fifth try, she said the house she sold to her parents and Lee reminded that she had sold the house but not to her parents. However, they had lived in the house after she sold it.

Then she started talking about her dad being all alone. Which was not so. He never lived alone. But she was adamant. It was fascinating to watch how she tried to make sense of her imperfect memories by embellishing with the words someone had just said or some piece of information from someplace else.

There was another interesting occurrence. After dinner, Jack rose from the table and went to his workroom and started looking at a catalog. This was not Jack's style. He would never leave company, no matter what. It was impolite. Through all our years together, he was always a hands-on host, making sure we had everything necessary for drinks and setting it up, making ice cubes, making sure there was a seat for every guest, making sure the closet had ample hangars and room for all the coats, pouring and refilling coffee cups, setting up, cleaning up.

Friday, March 17, 2006

We celebrated Tricia's birthday by taking her out for dinner and stopping to get an ice cream cake to enjoy in the evening. It was a day of grace. We all enjoyed dining out. There was calm and peace. A good day.

Saturday, March 18, 2006

After two weeks, the letter about the Mercury sticker resurfaced again. Jack is convinced that he has to take the car in and **they** won't do it and **they** will send him somewhere else. He spent the entire day agonizing over this and is preparing to take the car in tomorrow. While reading the labels with information on the proper way to set up the jack, he said, "I don't understand why my name is all over these."

Dear, Lord, this is breaking my heart. And how do I handle this? I don't want him to go alone because he can't communicate well. It will be embarrassing for him. I need to go with him. You know I'd rather not.

All evening long, it was on his mind and he kept making comments about being sent here and there. After several hours, he suddenly said, "I don't trust those bastards. I've been driving this car all the time. If I take it in, **they** will screw it up. After all, I don't go two hundred miles an hour."

Ah Ha! An out. "Jack, the car works fine. There is nothing wrong with it. The tires are fine." I added, "I think you are very smart to leave well enough alone." And that's where it stands for now. If I can get my hands on that packet of information, I am going to deep six it.

Saturday, March 25, 2006

Tricia went out with friends tonight. I always tell Jack where Tricia is going, but he doesn't remember. This evening he said, "I don't know where she is. You two talk and she goes off. If you crashed to the floor, how would I know where she is?" That gave me insight. His tone of voice belied a fear of being all alone and wondering how he would handle such a situation. I, too, wonder. Would he know what to do? Would he call 911? Does he remember what 911 is for? Would he be able to get the right words out?

Sunday, March 26, 2006
This afternoon, as Tricia and I were returning from a walk, we saw Jack outside talking with our landscaper. There is an area by the back porch that is quite barren. A decrepit evergreen was pulled out last year and the large stones around the porch were removed because they were cracking. Last spring Jack sowed grass seed. The summer saw very little rain and the grass died in the drought even with watering. The soil is like clay and the tender shoots couldn't survive the rock hard ground. In the fall, Jack sowed again, but nothing came up. He was puzzled and so was I until I realized that he had sown fertilizer instead of grass seed.

The landscaper suggested putting a small brick patio around the porch. It is a great idea. He will give us an estimate and bring brick samples in a few days. Jack was interested in the idea of a patio. I thought he would object to it because of cost. But he hasn't even mentioned the cost. Since the concept of money has eluded him more and more, I think the thought of what it would cost hasn't even crossed his mind.

Tuesday, March 28, 2006
For about a year now, the closet light has been kept on at night with the door partially closed. This gives enough light so the bedroom is not totally dark when we awaken in the middle of the night. This morning the light was not on when we woke up.

The fluorescent light over the vanity works off the same wall switch. It has been temperamental for some time. When Jack couldn't get the closet light to work by flipping the switch on and off and the fluorescent bulbs wouldn't light either, he was positive that the switch was broken. He dismissed my suggestion to replace the bulb in the closet to see if it was just burnt out.

As usual, he was fixated on the problem and didn't even finish his tea at breakfast. He was up and setting out for the bedroom with a screwdriver. I went down to the basement and brought up a ladder and a bulb. That's all it took and there was light in the closet.

Jack was still convinced that something was wrong with the outlet. He took off the plate and was going to poke around with the screwdriver. I cautioned that he shouldn't fool around until the power was turned off in the fuse box in the basement.

He said, "Turning something off downstairs isn't going to do anything up here."

"Yes, it would. It would keep you from being electrocuted. I don't want to see you hurt."

"I've been doing this for years. I know what I am doing."

"Yes. And for years you always turned the power off before doing something."

"Don't tell me what to do about something I've been doing for years!"

"You always turned the power off first. You always told me what an idiot that friend of yours was. He worked for the electric company. But he didn't turn the power off while working on the electricity at home and really gave himself a shock."

Round and round we went. This was one time when I would not back down for the sake of peace and quiet. Too much was at stake.

Finally, Jack said to me, "Go sit at your desk and read a book and let me be."

"I will. I am going to sit as close to the phone as possible, so when you electrocute yourself, I can dial 911 immediately."

Silence. Then, "You don't understand. But go ahead. Do what you want. I suppose you want to call an electrician?"

"I do." At last, a break in his refusal to call one because **they** would charge too much for nothing." The situation was defused (just noticed the pun).

Immediately, I found a referral in our local homeowners guide for an electrician who was recommended by neighbors. I called and by noon, he was here.

The switch in the bedroom was fine. The fluorescent bulbs were not. Both needed to be replaced.

Since he was here, I mentioned the switch in the garage which definitely was not fine. He went to inspect it and asked what happened as he surveyed the chipped paint and torn wallboard around it. I explained that when the ceiling light wouldn't stay on when Jack flipped the switch because it was loose, he would stabilize it with electrical tape. Every time he took the tape off to shut off the light, bits and pieces of wallboard and paint came with it.

The garage switch was definitely defective and actually illegal according to modern codes. Both switches in the box would have to be replaced. The second one was unusual because it was connected to three different outlets in the laundry room and kitchen. This was done efficiently.

The light over the table in the breakfast nook was also inspected and the wires properly attached and it, too, now works.

All the while the electrician was here, Jack would follow along to each different area of the house. As he walked, he was leaning more and more to the right just like he did when we were shopping at Christmas. It occurs when he is stressed. The more stressful the situation, the more he leans to the right. When the stress is really high, the degree of the angle is so pronounced he seems to be in danger of falling over. Amazing.

THEY LIVED AT OUR HOUSE

Thursday, March 30, 2006

A beautiful, sunny, warm day. The promise of days to come. After cleaning up the two flower beds along the front walkway, I measured out the area for the patio and marked it with stones. I showed Jack where the stones were so he could see what size the patio would be. He surveyed it placidly.

Once again, this is a bittersweet situation. It's sweet because we are in agreement like we used to be. It's bitter because the total absence of questions indicates how much destruction there is in that area of the brain.

Friday, March 31, 2006

The landscaper came by with the brick and Jack selected the caramel color which blends with the cedar siding. It pleases me that the artist's eye has not been diminished. The dimensions of the patio were also finalized.

Tonight Jack was getting ready to shower when I heard him call me. He had a tube of body lotion with the cap unscrewed. He said he couldn't figure out how to keep the lotion from running all over. I screwed the cap back on and flipped open the lid that covers the hole that the lotion comes out of when the tube is squeezed.

Looking around, I noticed that he did have a bath towel ready. This was good because the last few times, I wasn't sure what he used to dry himself off, since all the bath towels were stacked neatly on the shelf. Assumed he used a hand towel.

I pulled out the shampoo from the cabinet. He said he had shampoo and indicated the tube of body lotion. Several times I tried to explain the difference. He was positive that the lotion tube was what he always used.

These are not welcome signs. Together with some subtle changes in dress, they are disturbing. Until now, there have been no problems with personal hygiene.

Jack has always been fastidious about his clothes. He wears slacks, a shirt and a sport jacket under a top coat or raincoat to go grocery shopping. In warmer weather, a zippered jacket will replace the sports coat and top coat.

When working around the house on projects, he would wear items that I would have tossed eons ago. But he never went outside the house without changing clothes and being shaved and combed. In the midst of the grittiest projects, he would change clothes to go to the hardware store for the right pipe fitting or caulking or tool. Always.

Saturday, April 8, 2006
After a week of daily rain, the ground was finally dry enough for the patio to be put in. It took three days to bring the job to completion. It adds beauty to the yard.

I was scheduled to treat my friend Rose to a birthday lunch today, but rescheduled for next Saturday. I considered going, but Jack said, "What if **they** need something?" He is no longer comfortable on his own.

Saturday, April 15, 2006
Rose and I finally had lunch today. For the past three days I had to explain to Jack each day that lunch wasn't that day but Saturday. Today there was confusion and concern about where I was going. Just to the restaurant a few blocks away.

Later, Tricia told me that her dad kept looking at the clock and saying, "Why is she gone so long? Where did she go?"

When Rose dropped me off, she saw Jack out on the front lawn. She commented that Jack and her husband John were doing the same thing, going after the weeds. But I'll bet that John wasn't using disinfectant and glass cleaner instead of weed killer.

Sunday, April 16, 2006

Easter Sunday! Last night Jack went to bed at midnight. We were going to the Resurrection Mass at 6:30 a.m. He woke me up at 1:20 a.m., 2:09 a.m., 3:12 a.m., 4:10 a.m. Each time I suggested sleeping until 5. At that time, he was dressed but sounding tired. I suggested going to a later Mass. He laid down but was up at 5:45 a.m.

Meanwhile I had dressed since sleep was a lost cause. So as dawn glimmered through last night's rain, we set out for Resurrection Mass. This was the first time Mass was being celebrated in the renovated church. That has created some new problems. Our short old pew is gone. There are very long ones. We sat in one closest to our old spot. When leaving the pew to receive Communion, there are now two steps to walk down. I was behind Jack and steadied him when he faltered. This is going to be a weekly problem unless we sit elsewhere. We'll have to find a better pew next week.

After breakfast, Jack was exhausted and I tucked him into bed. He was asleep as soon as his head touched the pillow. I sat down in the living room for a moment and nodded off myself.

As usual, Jack's sisters were invited for Easter dinner. Without the doll business to worry about and no production to complete, it was a joy making the holiday preparations. On Saturday, everything was done except for the last minute dishes. Put the ham in the oven, unmold the gelatin, cut the bread, fix the green bean casserole and the coffeepot and that was it.

Jack's sisters were expected at 3 p.m. They didn't arrive until after 4 p.m. LaVerne couldn't find her keys. She said she left them at church. That wasn't possible because she had to use the car key to drive home and the house key to get in the front door. But she did not put the keys in the lock on the inside of the door. Both sisters searched the house for an hour without success. When they finally left the house, it was raining and the drive was not easy.

THEY LIVED AT OUR HOUSE

The decline in LaVerne is apparent. The always impeccable, stylish, well put together woman is no longer. Her clothes are okay. She still wears heels and jewelry. Lee said that she has worn the same outfit wherever she goes. A big change for a woman with eighty-four blouses in her closet.

Most noticeable is the decline in perfection. Its lack showed in her makeup and definitely in her hair. It needs washing, combing, styling. No longer haute couture head to toe.

Monday, April 17, 2006

The keys are still missing. Another search through the house did not find the keys. However, while looking for them, LaVerne opened a drawer in a highboy in the bedroom and there were her eyeglasses, the ones she lost last summer!

The only recourse was to go and get new keys. The local hardware store had blanks for the house key but not for the car. A new key would have to be obtained from the dealership.

It cost thirty dollars for the new key. LaVerne balked at the price. Lee muttered, "Pay it." So she did. And they went home.

When they reached the house, LaVerne did not have the key. This triggered a search of LaVerne's purse, her coat pockets, the car. No key. The dealership was called. The key were not left on the counter.

So it was back for another key which had to be driven over from another dealership. LaVerne did not wait patiently. When the key arrived, the manager put it on a distinctive key ring and gave it to LaVerne without cost. After all her impatience, he was eager to get her out of the showroom.

LaVerne would not cooperate when Lee tried to organize the keys she had into a set to be used, an extra set and spare keys. "I will do what I want to do. Stop bossing me!" She kept mixing up the keys. It was an impossible task and Lee finally left at wit's end. As Lee related this story to me, she was emotionally bereft. How I empathized with her as I know the feeling all too well. So do all other caregivers of those with dementia.

It is a human need to want to be thanked after expending extraordinary time and effort doing something for someone. It is very hard to accept the vitriolic words one often receives instead. Thank You is the balm that soothes the exhausted soul and reenergizes it.

But dementia causes its victim's mind to lose sight of the needs and wants of others. It is not done with malice as it sometimes looks. It is done with the same innocence of the baby whose simple mind can only focus on itself. The mind affected by dementia is too busy trying to hang on to its independence. When someone is accustomed to putting herself first, getting appreciation is a lost cause.

In our conversation I also learned that LaVerne no longer drives to her sister's house. It is a short easy run that she has done thousands of times over many years. But the last time she tried driving back to her own home, she could not remember how. Apparently she stopped at a business to ask directions and the person at the desk recognized her confusion and called the police. One of the policemen drove LaVerne home in her car while the other followed in the squad car.

LaVerne was absolutely astonished to learn that everyone knows she has a problem. She accused us of gossiping about her and was told that no one had to say anything. Neighbors and friends and people she knows at her church were asking what was wrong.

We both agree that the time has come to set in motion plans for LaVerne to move to a facility where she will receive the care she needs. Any mention of a live-in caregiver or someone who would come several days a week has been met with anger and absolute refusal. She doesn't want anyone in her house and she is not going anywhere. She'd rather commit suicide first. This has stopped her sister from taking any action.

LaVerne will not go quietly. She will go ballistic when she learns of our intent. We will have to make all the plans. We will have to have everything in place and tell her only at the very last possible minute.

At present, I am needed here 24/7 and will have to figure out a way to help with all the arrangements without too many trips to the western suburbs.

I volunteered to be the fall guy since it is necessary for Lee to be in good graces since she is handling her affairs and will see her many more times than I will. If LaVerne is going to be angry, let it be directed at me as the instigator.

All her life, LaVerne has focused on the things of this world and of what value are they to her now? Nothing matters. The statue that she guarded so solicitously on a return trip from Europe because she paid a great price for it now stands with a broken arm. And she laughs it off because she no longer knows the value or cares. All those years of delight in her possessions are gone like so much chaff in the wind.

My poor Jack. He never sought after material things. His interests were in reading and art. Now, too, all that knowledge so laboriously gained is lost.

Dear God, I know You have reasons why this brother and sister are afflicted in this way. My heart breaks for both of them. I give these two people so dear to my heart into Your Hands for safekeeping.

Tuesday, April 18, 2006

LaVerne called early this morning. She was laughing. "The funniest thing happened. I lost my keys yesterday and my sister came and we looked all over the house and couldn't find them.

"We had to go to the car dealer to get a new one. I paid for it. This dumb girl gave me the receipt but she never gave me the key. So we had to go back. She left it on the counter.

"This morning I was making my bed. You know that chest that I have by the foot of the bed? The keys were caught up in the bedspread!"

Thursday, April 20, 2006

After working with rock and edging all day, a hot and sweaty me was desperately in need of a relaxing bath and a good washing of hair. Just finished washing my hair, when Tricia came inside and said, "Mom, you'd better go outside. Daddy is putting dandruff shampoo on the bare spots in the lawn."

This was not a grass guru's concoction for a beautiful lawn. This was forgetting what lawn products to use. It does make my imagination take off. If it rains tonight, instead of Kentucky blue grass, will we have bubbly blue grass in the morning? That makes me laugh. I choose to laugh. If I don't laugh, I'll cry.

Tuesday, April 25, 2006

Another worry. I walked into the powder room because I saw an ant on the carpet. Noticed that the rug was lumpy behind the toilet. Bent down to flatten the rug. The rug was fine. It was the floor underneath that was lumpy. Touched the rug to pull it back and it was wet. So were the floorboards underneath. The corner of one board was warped from water.

Just what I don't need. The toilet seal is probably broken and water has been seeping out each time the commode is used. It's probably been going on for quite a while but wasn't obvious because the carpet has been absorbing all the water. The flooring will have to be replaced which means removing the toilet. I don't know if it can be reseated. It and the sink are an odd color of peachy beige. That color went out of style years ago.

Cautioned Tricia not to use the powder room but I won't say anything to Jack just yet. He will want to fix it himself and that is out of the question. I need to talk to a few people who might give me some helpful information on how to handle this.

Sunday, April 30, 2006

It is Sunday and Jack did not wake me until 6 a.m. It was amazing. At breakfast, he said to me "I can't understand it. I was trying to figure out the time and my dad said to me, 'If you get up at five, you will have plenty of time.' I don't understand because..." His voice trailed off.

I'm rearranging my workroom so I can move the computer. It will free up space in Jack's art room. I'd like to bring up one of the easels. Maybe if he could paint, it might be therapeutic for him. He hasn't painted on canvas in so long, I don't know what will happen. But it is worth a try.

He hasn't been able to read for a long time because he can't retain what is read. Watching television is becoming a problem because everything is so fast paced and it is hard for him to follow the story line. He can no longer putter in the basement and fix the things that need repair because those skills are also gone.

Tuesday, May 9, 2006

Moved the computer into my workroom this morning. Once it was out of his room, Jack eagerly cleaned up his drawing board and artist's tabaret and the file cabinet top. With nothing on the drawing board, we were able to move it away from the windows so I could wash them. They had been impossible to reach and needed a good cleaning for a long time. Also cleaned the shutters, baseboards and fixtures. When all was done we rearranged the drawing board so it is more efficient.

This evening I stopped by to see the neighbor who is a remodeling contractor. He works on major renovations. I hoped that he could give me the name of someone who would fix the powder room floor. He said he has done it before and would be happy to do it.

I explained that I did not want to get into a situation that would be too stressful for Jack. I wanted the easiest solution possible. He said the current toilet could probably be reseated. It is tricky because of its age. Oftentimes, they crack.

He said he would come by on Monday or Tuesday to assess the damage to the floor. He would bring catalogs I could refer to if I chose replacement of the sink cabinet as well. He said it would take a day to replace the floor, about four days to do a total replacement.

Sunday, May 14, 2006

On this Mother's Day, I asked Jack's mom to look after her little boy. If she were still on earth, how devastated she would be to see him this way. We had a quiet dinner of turkey, fresh corn on the cob, salad, green beans and fruit compote.

Since our neighbor was coming by tomorrow or Tuesday to assess the damage in the bathroom, I mentioned the leak so Jack would not be taken by surprise. Immediately, he tried to get into the crawl space to see if the water was dripping down there. He couldn't get the light to work and had a difficult time climbing in and out of the crawl space.

Monday, May 15, 2006

Jack was up bright and early. He found a light that worked well and climbed back into the crawl space. Then he wanted to go to Home Depot to see what he could get to fix the floor. He ignored my comments that it would be a complicated job. He and his dad put in toilets in the house where he grew up. It wasn't hard. No recall that that was over fifty years ago.

Wednesday, May 17, 2006

The powder room is filling Jack with apprehension. He transfers his worry about that to every other aspect of life. The negative attitude is such a killer to live with. It seems like the Alzheimer's disease has ravaged the parts of his brain that focused on the good and left those parts that only remember the bad.

All the literature on Alzheimer's Disease promotes focusing on memories from long ago as a good way of providing calm and peace to the person with Alzheimer's. As the person moves into the stages of Alzheimer's, these are usually the last memories to disappear. It sounds great, but it doesn't work with Jack. No matter what occasion I mention, he responds with a negative comment. If I mention the beautiful sunsets on Sanibel Island, he'll bring up the sunburn on his legs from walking the beach. If the topic is a restaurant we used to enjoy, he'll focus on the one time there was a long wait or service was slow.

Thursday, May 18, 2006

Called the contractor today and told him Jack was straining at the bit. If he could just give me a referral, I would appreciate it. He promised that he would be here on Saturday at 10 a.m. He was finishing off another job and would be free once the job was completed.

In the afternoon, we needed a change of pace. Jack and I went to the garden center to buy geraniums and dusty miller to edge the walkways. We made two trips to buy the twenty bags of red mulch needed around the flowers. The trunk will only hold ten bags at one time.

The walkways look beautiful with peach geraniums and silvery dusty miller intermingled with the light yellow-green leaves of euonymous and all highlighted by the background of red cedar mulch.

Saturday, May 20, 2006

Jack was up and dressed before 6 a.m., even though the contractor wouldn't be coming until 10:30. I decided to leave the situation fully in God's Hands. If the contractor only mentioned replacing the floor and reseating the toilet, okay. When he came, he resolved the issue by tearing out the toilet and the flooring assuming that I was going to do it all.

We discussed the basics that would be needed. He said he would pick out what he thought would work and show it to me. He would bring samples of countertops and flooring, He gave me brochures on the various styles of cabinets that would fit in the available space. He knew I couldn't traipse from store to store picking things out as most people do.

So the die is cast. The powder room will be remodeled. I hope all goes well.

Sunday, May 21, 2006

More slippage is occurring. The other day Tricia noticed her dad was wearing a pair of my jeans. This morning he couldn't understand what was wrong with his cold cereal. He put salt on it instead of artificial sweetener.

We all do weird things. But we realize that we made a mistake and how it happened. That's what is missing in a person with Alzheimer's. They know something is wrong or lost or missing or awry. But they are no longer capable of figuring out why and what to do to rectify the situation.

Friday, May 26, 2006

Jack was ready to go grocery shopping at 5:30 a.m. this morning. I mentioned that the stores don't open until 7 a.m. He was upset. He is concerned that the contractor's trucks will block him from getting out of the garage.

THEY LIVED AT OUR HOUSE

Going to the grocery store is a good activity for him. He walks around slowly looking at everything. He no longer rushes to get a gallon of milk before I am halfway through the store. Now I usually need to remind him to select a gallon. He has become much more passive in his involvement in daily activity.

While at store, we found two good looking steaks to grill at dinnertime. It is an activity that has been solely his through our married life. I have never gone near the grill except to hand him a plate of meat or veggies when the fire is ready. Jack had no trouble starting the fire and cooking the steaks to perfection.

While I cleaned up the dishes, he went out to put the charcoal grill away. I wondered why I didn't see the charcoal can on the patio. He uses a large popcorn tin to store used charcoal. He pours the used coals into the popcorn tin, covers it tightly and the coals die out. Jack was on the driveway pouring water into the tin of hot coals. The mucky water was seeping through the seams in the tin and running down the driveway.

Monday, May 29, 2006

Memorial Day! Dear Lord, you know how I wish I could be unfailingly patient with everyone. What a trying day!

The morning was busy preparing for Jack's sisters to come for a cookout. The day was a humid and hot 90°. Jack could not understand why the men were not here to work on the powder room. Holidays have little deep meaning for him. He no longer remembers when he savored these respites from daily work. Now one day is no different from any other day.

In the afternoon, just before his sisters were due to arrive, I saw Jack walking down the hall to the bedroom with the bottle of whiskey in one hand and a small shot glass in the other. I asked him why he was taking the whiskey to the bedroom. He said he needed it for his eyes. I replied, "You can't put liquor in your eyes. You will hurt them."

He launched into a fifteen-minute diatribe. "I have to put 'this' in 'there' at 'that time', but not 'then' because I listened to what the doctor said. I have to do it or I'll be done for. You don't know what's going on because you don't listen but I do and I know what I am doing. The next time I go to the doctor I am going to tell him that you are interfering. I've been doing this since I was in Korea and it'll be your fault if I go blind...." on and on and on. All the while he was banging the bottle and the shot glass together until I was sure one would break.

Tears formed in my eyes as I watched this stranger who used to be my gentle husband. I could feel myself deflating inwardly with depression. The feeling was momentary as I realized that it didn't matter what he said as long as a mishap or tragedy was averted or a course of behavior was altered.

The verbal explosion left Jack exhausted and forgetful of what he intended to do with the whiskey and glass. He put them on the countertop in the kitchen where he always sets up the necessities for drinks. He assumed the role of bartender from the very beginning of our marriage and would never relinquish it. Today he probably was setting out the ice and whiskey and glasses when he had a thought about putting eye drops in his eyes and his thought processes got muddled up.

Inwardly, I was still a bit shaken when Lee and LaVerne arrived a few minutes later. They brought charcoal for the grill and I carried it out back. Jack had the old yellow cooker on the patio. The charcoal trays were warped and would not sit properly in the bottom of the cooker. He pulled them out and was going to dump the charcoal directly into the bottom of the cooker. Again, it was difficult to convince him that there were holes in the bottom through which ash and embers would fall out.

I wondered if his blood glucose was low and triggering so much faulty thinking and agitation. He would not come into the house, so I brought the glucometer outside but he would not take a reading.

After what seemed like eons, he was convinced that he could cook four burgers on the small grill. I took the yellow grill back to the garage and brought out the small portable picnic one. As the situation calmed down, everyone settled on the patio and I served cool drinks and shrimp. As I went to sit down on a folding lawn chair, it collapsed inwardly inviting my nose to touch my knees. Did the chair understand how I felt?

On such a hot day, the charcoal was ready in no time. Jack had calmed down and was able to tend to the burgers without a problem. I noticed that once again he was leaning to the right a bit as he walked, a sign of stress.

The grilled hamburgers were delicious and we all enjoyed a typical summer cookout with fresh fruit, potato salad and corn on the cob. We ate a bit early which turned out to be a blessing.

At 5 p.m. the sky darkened, the winds revved up and a huge storm poured down rain. Since it came from the west, the patio and porch stayed dry.

After all the earlier turmoil, I did lose my patience with LaVerne. She came into the kitchen while I was putting the leftover salads in savers and cleaning up the dishes.

"My sister is always telling me what to do. It's not fair. She knows everything. Nothing is wrong with her. But I have this damn disease. Why do I have to have it?"

"LaVerne, we all have problems. Lee has hers, too."

"She doesn't have any problems."

"Yes, she does. She just doesn't talk about them."

"All my life, it was good. I never worried. I was healthy."

"How lucky you were not to have problems for so many years. Many people have them all their lives."

"But you don't understand. It's not fair to start having problems at my age." She launched into her tirade about God and widows.

I couldn't take another minute of the same old tirades.

"LaVerne, I don't want to hear that again." I walked away.

Tuesday, May 30, 2006

When we had the patio put in last month, our good neighbor offered his van to pick up a patio set. I put off doing anything about it during the days of cold, rainy weather. Last week, when I called the store that had the one I liked, they were sold out. I had hoped to have it for the holiday yesterday.

Today, the store manager called and said a new shipment had come in. After dinner my neighbor drove me over to the store. Jack was asleep when I left. When he awoke he kept asking Tricia where I was, if I ate, when I was coming back, why was it taking so long, etc. etc. Knowing how he is about my being out of his sight, it worked well that he was asleep when I left.

We returned home and our neighbor carried the large box to the back porch. Jack did not recognize him. He thought he was a delivery man. More decline.

Wednesday, May 31, 2006

This morning was spent putting the patio chairs together. What a reversal of roles. I did the unpacking of the parts and the putting together, the work Jack always did. He disposed of the cardboard, plastic wrap and other packing materials, which had always been my job.

By trial and error, I learned how to use hex wrenches. At first, I wondered why two were enclosed in the package. Soon realized I needed one to hold the bolt steady while the other one screwed on the nut.

Amazingly, Jack never said a word that I was doing it wrong and didn't know what I was doing. He was a passive bystander who was very helpful. It was so odd. He never said, "I should be doing that" or "Let me do it." Yet, he did go down to the basement and bring up a set of enclosed hex wrenches that he remembered he had.

When we finally found the right sizes to use, what a huge difference it made. It took me forty-five minutes to do the first chair. A half hour for the second. With the right hex wrenches, it only took fifteen minutes each for the remaining two chairs. After lunch, we tackled the table. Tricia held the legs to the support until I had all the screws started. All the pieces were up and functional by 3 p.m. It is the right size set for our patio. The chair cushions are soft. The bases swivel and rock. We ate pizza out on the patio. It was lovely. The cloudiness of the day decreased. The sky was deep blue with puffs of white. The foliage is a vibrant spring green with touches of color. All in all, a very good day. Thank You, God.

Thursday, June 1, 2006

The fixtures have been pulled out of the powder room and the floor underlayment is being done. The new cabinet has been ordered and should be delivered in a few days. The countertop will take much longer since it is not a stock item and has to be specially made. I ordered a silver framed mirror which will be a wonderful complement to the blue selected for the walls.

Saturday, June 3, 2006

Jack has been calm the past few days. I considered going out for dinner, just the two of us. Menus have become hard to read and understand. The restaurant we like has their menu on line. I ran a copy off and gave it to Jack. It was confusing.

Home is the perfect restaurant. No driving to and fro, inattentive wait staff, loud patrons, bills and tips to calculate. We had baked potatoes, lobster tails and salad on sectioned plates. We toasted each other with sparkling wine. For dessert, there were eclairs and tea. All the while, we enjoyed the blue skies and gentle breezes while sitting on the new patio set.

It was a perfect evening. Jack was relaxed. Nothing was upsetting him. He reminisced for a long time while I listened and watched the new moon gradually traverse the deepening blue of the eastern sky. In the background were the gentle melodies of the rustling leaves.

If only for the memories of this lovely night with a peaceful Jack, I would have paid a million dollars for the patio.

Friday, June 9, 2006

The past week has been relatively uneventful, for which I am most grateful. I know it won't last for long. But I thank God for letting me have time to recharge my batteries for whatever the future holds.

Sunday, June 11, 2006

At 6 a.m. this morning, Jack was up. I thought, "Good, he slept all through the night and is waking up at the right time for Sunday Mass." However, when I touched him I could feel the telltale dampness of skin that heralds a hypoglycemic reaction. His blood glucose was 55. He ate breakfast. I tucked him back into bed. He was cold and tired.

I decided the Red Letter Day had come. Tricia and I dressed for church. Since Jack was sleeping, I left a note for him should he awaken. I drove to church. For the first time in eons.

When we returned home Jack was still asleep. Later in the day I told him we had gone to church. He accepted it as quietly as when he relinquished the checkbook last year.

Monday, June 12, 2006

This morning we needed to have our prescriptions filled. I called them in to the local pharmacy. In the afternoon when Jack awoke, I said that I was going to pick them up. He accepted the fact placidly.

Tricia and I went together. As we drove along, she looked at me with wonder in her eyes. I reminded her of all the times in the past when she would say, "Mom, you have your license. You should drive." At those times any suggestion of doing such a thing would have triggered agitation in her dad. I would tell her, "The time will come. Be patient."

The time has come without trauma and disregard for Jack's self esteem. Praise be to God! All things in His time.

Tuesday, June 13, 2006

Over the weekend, Jack was tending to his feet and nicked his toe. Tricia noticed him running back and forth to get adhesive bandages. Today he let me look at the toe. Definitely, his foot needs professional attention and I called for an appointment with a podiatrist. The best I could schedule was nine days from today. Most of these doctors have multiple offices so they are only in the area one or two days a week. It seems like a long time but should be okay as long as the toe doesn't get worse.

Friday, June 16, 2006

Jack will not leave his toe alone. He keeps soaking it and trying to dig under the thickened nail. It is not looking better. I am concerned because his foot is cool to the touch which means circulation is not good. That is critical to the healing of the cut.

Every night we are up at the oddest hours. His appetite is been declining and he has refused most foods. This results in hypoglycemic reactions. The toe is bothersome. He is restless. By 5 a.m. he is exhausted. After an early breakfast, I will tuck him in under the warm covers and he will sleep through the morning.

Meanwhile, I dress and wait for the workmen to come at 7:30 a.m. On Wednesday, the electrician put in can lights in the soffit and the carpenter started putting in the floor, not an easy task judging by the mumbling under his breath.

On Thursday, Jack slept until noon through all the pounding and hammering and the din of a boom box set to soft rock. The men are working in a tight area that is hot because of the small room size and the work is tedious. They did a great job leveling the floor by building up the concrete base for the tiles so the toilet will be seated properly.

Saturday, June 17, 2006

Jack's toe is not healing. It is starting to discolor which is not a good sign. I tried to call other doctors without success since it is Saturday. I was sitting on the patio talking on the phone with Frank when Jack came out in a panic. "I've got to get something done." I told him the only thing we could do was go to the emergency room. That caused great agitation. When he calmed down a bit, he still adamantly refused to go today. He said he would go tomorrow.

Sunday, June 18, 2006

Jack was up on and off all night. Neither of us had much sleep. It began to rain in the morning before we were ready to leave for church. Jack said he couldn't find his car keys which I knew were in his pocket. He would not let me check his pockets and he wouldn't do so either. He insisted I had them and wanted to search my purse, which I would not let him do. He started talking about "going there and sitting in the car with all the other cars and no one knowing what to do and then they walked out and told everybody to go without getting anything done...." He was not making sense.

I would not let him drive to church. He refused to let me do so. It was best not to go. Standing would be hard on his foot. The Mass is always a source of great comfort to me each week. But under the circumstances, there was no other option. Prayer can be done anywhere.

Jack was exhausted after the outburst and slept until noon. When he awoke, he refused to go to the emergency room. He said he would wait until morning. I could get an appointment for him on Monday.

The all day rain certainly put a damper on Father's Day cookouts. Of course, the day was just another day to Jack. I fixed his favorite dinner. He was surprised when I set the plate before him. But he ate it with gusto. This is in sharp contrast to most of his meals during the past few months. He has been eating less and less. He says that some foods choke him. I wonder if the Alzheimer's is beginning to annihilate the parts of the brain that control the signals governing chewing and swallowing.

In the evening while watching TV, Jack suddenly said to me, "He hasn't been here, has he?"

I asked, "Who?"

"You know, they...God."

"God?"

"No, not God. You know, them, yours and mine."

"You mean our parents?" my intuition prompted.

"Yes. Well, I know mine weren't."

"Well, neither have mine. They've been gone a long time."

Monday, June 19, 2006

Jack was up at 4 a.m. wanting to know if I had gotten an appointment for him. After 9 a.m., I finally found a podiatrist who would see him this afternoon.

The doctor looked at the toe and said that it appeared to be caught in time. The it being infection and gangrene. He checked the reflexes on the soles of Jack's feet. There were none, not a good sign. He prodded different areas of the foot and kept asking if Jack felt anything. The tops of his feet still have feeling.

The soles are definitely neuropathic. In part, this may be why he has been able to withstand the pain. Since the foot is not normal, he does not feel as much pain. It also explains why his shoes do not feel good and why he is so unsure of himself when he walks. If he can't feel where his foot really is because the sole is not picking up the signal through the damaged nerve endings, it could cause the unsteady gait.

Jack was told that it would take six to eight weeks for the toe to heal. If it looks worse in the next two days, we should call the podiatrist or contact Jack's physician. He would have to be hospitalized. He used a salve on the toe to draw out blood and detritus. An antibiotic was prescribed to help prevent further infection.

I drove home with unsolicited advice from the passenger seat. I reminded Jack that he had been driving nonstop for over fifty years. I haven't, but I felt very comfortable behind the wheel. Fortunately, his comments do not rattle me at all. When I get behind the wheel, my mind switches into a different mode: this is how I am driving, safely and sanely, and nothing will make me deviate from that goal.

We stopped at the pharmacy to pick up the antibiotic, salve, gauze and tape to rewrap the toe each day after cleaning it and putting on the salve. All was calm.

The minute we walked into the house, Jack began a tirade against "that guy." All afternoon. All evening. "He doesn't know what he is doing. It's a scheme. **They** set this up. **They** think **they** can fool me. I know what I am doing. I've been dealing with this since Korea. Nothing like that happened then. I'll give him one or two more times but I don't like it. It's all a moneymaking scheme. **They** don't know what **they** are doing. If **they** try something, I'll flatten them."

Tuesday, June 20, 2006

Jack woke up in an agitated state. He came walking down the hallway dragging the brown comforter. He complained that his feet were freezing, the bedroom was too cold and he wasn't going to sleep there. When I walked into the bedroom, the whole bed was a shambles. The other comforter was hanging off, the top sheet was all tangled up on one side of the bed. Everything was awry.

His feet are cool to the touch because of poor circulation. He has complained about that for a while but would go ballistic if I mentioned having it checked out by his vascular surgeon. Until he suddenly decided that he needed to get something done for his toe because it was starting to turn black and blue.

He was up at all hours of the night thinking he should be somewhere. That's the current pattern. Up on and off all night, breakfast early in the morning, then sleeping like a log until noon or so. Nothing bothers him when he is asleep in the morning. The workmen sawing, drilling, pounding. He will sleep through everything.

The powder room is coming along nicely. The drywall is almost finished. Tomorrow it will be sanded and primed. I can paint the room before the cabinet and toilet are put in.

God certainly knows what he is doing. Initially, I viewed the leaking toilet as the last thing I needed at this stressful time in our lives. But it has turned out to be a blessing. It has given me something else to think about. Otherwise, my mind would be totally preoccupied with the depressingly rapid declines in Jack and dread of what the future holds for him.

Jack awoke around 1 p.m. He refused lunch and took up where he had left off yesterday, railing about **they** and what **they** think **they** are doing, on and on. I let him get some of it out of his system, then reminded him that the medication was to help heal his foot. If he wanted me to put it on, I would soak his foot, dry it, put on the salve and a fresh dressing. Just let me know. I left it at that. It worked. He grew quiet and was very cooperative through the whole procedure.

I wish I knew how his brain is perceiving things. The visit to the podiatrist had to be confusing. Everything happens much too quickly for a brain that isn't whole. Small wonder that what is said makes no sense.

For dinner I served beef and corn and pineapple, the only fruit that he hasn't refused to eat. Forget the nutrition charts. I no longer care about what he should or should not eat because he is diabetic or should watch his sodium intake. I am grateful when I can get him to eat any amount of food.

Thursday, June 22, 2006

This morning, while tending to Jack's foot, I found two ulcerated areas beneath the fourth and fifth toes on the underside of the foot. Taking him to the emergency room was the only option. Fortunately, he did not rebel against the decision.

When we arrived at the entrance to the emergency room, there were no empty parking spaces. I wanted to leave him in the car and go to get a volunteer who would help him while I parked the car elsewhere. Jack did not want me to do that. He said we should park in the lot near the north pavilion. I hesitated to do so because it is quite a walk from the parking lot to the entrance. He insisted. Not wanting to initiate any refusal to enter the hospital, I drove over.

The lot was full except for one spot that looked too small. I didn't think that I could maneuver the car into the spot. My sight isn't as accurate as Jack's is. He looked directly at me and said, "You can do it." I did. And we both walked slowly from the lot to the hospital entrance.

Once inside the lobby, I made a beeline for the reception desk and asked for directions to the emergency room. (I knew the way. I really needed a wheelchair. But if I had asked for one,

Jack would have been upset.) The fellow behind the desk jumped up, assessed the situation, secured a wheelchair, settled Jack in it and set off at a brisk pace for the ER before Jack knew what was happening.

Once there, a volunteer took over and wheeled Jack to a desk where a nurse asked why we were there. She looked at Jack's foot and immediately began calling floors to determine bed availability.

From there we were whisked to cubicle seven where a small army of nurses, technicians and the ER doctor marched in and out. They drew blood, checked blood pressure and temperature, took chest X-rays, examined the foot and did a Doppler on the leg to determine circulation. When the Doppler was done, I, too, heard the absence of sound. Blood was not flowing well through the veins. The technician and doctor looked at each other. I knew what that look meant. The doctor told the nurse that they would need to call in a vascular surgeon. I mentioned the name of the one Jack had seen several years previously. The ER doctor was relieved that staff would not have to call around.

Through all of this Jack was calm. He sat placidly, with a little smile on his face, almost like a teddy bear. He was taken to four north, which is the pulmonary floor. However, the young fellow in the room with him had had surgery on his leg. The nurses settled him in and ordered a dinner tray. He ate a little but not much. I didn't worry because I knew the staff would be monitoring his blood glucose and would tend to it if it fell too low. For all his dementia, he was still thoughtful and kept offering his food to me. I was not hungry. The nurses would also monitor his food intake and the amount needed to be accurate.

All the while Jack was still calm. Before I left, I told him that I would call him when I arrived at home. He beat me to it. I had just walked in the door when the phone rang. A nurse had dialed the number for Jack. He was worried that it had taken too long for me to drive the few miles between hospital and home.

Around midnight, I was getting ready to wash my hair and take a quick bath. The phone rang and the nightmare began. The nurses at the desk on four north were calling. They asked if I had any difficulty with Jack at night. He was agitated. Perhaps if I spoke to him, it would help. I said that I would call the room. The nurse said that he would give the phone to Jack who was standing at the door of his room.

When Jack took the phone, I asked him what the problem was. He said, "I need the forty-foot ladders and I need ..... unintelligible..." The phone dropped. I could hear him shouting. Someone tried to steady him and he shouted, "Get your hands off me or I'll flatten you."

Another nurse picked up the phone. She said that they had given him a sleeping pill at 10 p.m., but it had no effect. She said Jack would not stay in bed. She wanted to know if I objected to the use of a posey restraint, a cloth device that prevents a person from getting out of bed. I told her that I would prefer that it not be used. But I understood the need to remember the welfare of all the other patients on the floor who were trying to sleep. If that was the only way...

Earlier in the evening, when I spoke to my brother, he said, "Well, you'll finally get a good night's sleep." So much for that. My mind is reeling. All I can think of is Jack. How I feel for him. How confused he must be. And how he must feel that I have abandoned him.

Friday, June 23, 2006

A catastrophic day. The nurse called around 8 a.m. to say that they had moved Jack to another room. An IV had been started in the emergency room yesterday and after the midnight episode they had given him a sedative through it. He slept and was drowsy all morning. Not much different from his current patterning at home.

Around 8:30 a.m., I went to the grocery store to pick up a few needed items. While I was there, Tricia called my cell and told me the nurses had called again.

Around 10 a.m., the vascular surgeon called. He had assessed Jack. He noted that Jack had tried to think about the questions asked, but would give the wrong answers. He said there was gangrene in the affected foot. His circulation was very poor. There was a good pulse at the knee. Of the three arteries traversing down the leg, only the inside one was okay and was probably feeding into the middle artery. The top artery which feeds the ankle and downward was blocked off. The forefoot was most seriously blocked. He could not hear any blood flow. An antibiotic was being used to keep the infection under control. The toe would have to be removed at the minimum.

The real question was that at some point a decision must be made to do an angiogram to see if an amputation below the knee could be avoided. Unfortunately, all of this can cause worsening of the mental functioning.

In diabetes, the sensory nerves become compromised. This results in neuropathy. It creates a problem with proprioception, awareness of space. There was a poor prognosis, no matter what was or wasn't done. It's like a house of playing cards. Once one is disturbed, others fall.

Just removing the toe would require several weeks of bed rest. The night before raised the question of Jack's understanding that he could not get out of bed. There was a good possibility that he might lose the ability to walk. He concluded by saying that he would schedule an angiogram for Monday, so it is on the books, since kidney function is normal. He said that the normal kidney function was a big surprise after forty years as a diabetic. The weekend will give Jack a chance to be stabilized. After the angiogram, all doctors involved would enter into a decision to revascularize to save the foot or amputate below the knee. My poor Jack!

While hanging up with the vascular surgeon, the neurologist called. She had assessed Jack and stated unequivocally that all the tests indicated that he had Alzheimer's Disease. No surprise there.

It was already after 11 a.m. and I still had to do the banking and a few other errands to prepare for the unknown that lay ahead. By the time they were accomplished, it was after 1 p.m. I grabbed a quick sandwich and set off for the hospital. Just as I arrived at the new room, the aides came in to help Jack out of bed and put him on a gurney. They were taking him to radiology for an ultrasound of the carotid arteries. I hugged him and told him I would be waiting for him when he returned.

I settled into a chair with a book of jokes and cartoons. I needed a bit of humor to deflate the stress balloon. I surmised that Jack had been placed in this room to minimize the disruption and noise for the rest of the patients. It is the first room as you leave the elevator lobby. In itself it is very quiet, being free of the usual hospital sounds from further down the floor.

I was about three minutes into the humor book when an ear shattering cough erupted from the man sharing the room. He looks about ninety years old, but he is still substantial in stature with a fringe of white hair and a somewhat sunken mouth. He was perfectly still. But every few minutes another loud cough would emanate from his throat.

A nurse came in to speak with him. He bellowed, "WHAT? I CAN'T HEAR YOU." (That was obvious.) "I DON'T HAVE MY HEARING AIDS AND I CAN'T FIND MY WALLET AND NO ONE KNOWS I'M HERE." Now I knew for sure why he and Jack were both in the same room.

The ultrasound completed, Jack was brought back to the room about ninety minutes later. He was tired and would start nodding off. Then the man's coughing would jolt him awake.

Around 4 p.m. the man's wife and granddaughter came to visit. "OH HAPPY DAY!" he shouted. "YOU CAME TO SEE

ME." His wife told him she brought his hearing aids. Then proceeded a half hour in which they would put the aid in one ear or the other and ask him if he could hear. "WHAT?" Which ear was better.? "I CAN'T HEAR WHAT YOU ARE SAYING."

At one point, his wife said, "Don't be so loud. There's a man in the other bed and he's trying to rest." He replied, "WELL TELL HIM THAT I LOVE HIM." That made me chuckle.

Amidst all of the din, I heard chimes playing a few chords of Brahm's *Lullaby*. I looked up at the TV, thinking it was a commercial. A baseball game was being televised. When an aide came into the room, she said that the chimes come over the loudspeaker every time a baby is born. What a wonderful idea! It is therapy for all. For staff who may be dealing with traumatic issues of the moment, patients who may be depressed and worried about their health, and visitors distressed at the ills affecting their loved ones. Immediately, I said a prayer for the newborn child with his or her whole life ahead. What will the little one's life be like? How long? With what will it be filled? Life goes on, thanks be to God.

The contents of Jack's dinner tray had been decided by staff the night before. He wouldn't eat the mostaccioli. An egg salad sandwich was brought up. He wouldn't eat that. Remembering last night when he kept trying to give me his food, I had gone down to the cafeteria before dinner and brought up some fish and a salad. We would have dinner together or so I hoped. He would only eat the pineapple and drink some of the milk. Neither of us ate much.

As soon as the trays were removed, he tried to get out of bed. He had the posey restraint on. I tried to calm him down, but couldn't. Neither could the nurses. He was so agitated, they put on hand restraints. It only exacerbated his agitation which was killing my heart.

"Go to the kitchen and get a knife," he kept saying as he struggled.

"There is no kitchen here. We are not at home. We are in the hospital."

"Go to the kitchen. Get a knife."

"Jack, please. If you will lay still, you will be freed from the restraints."

"I don't believe you would do this to me. Making a fool out of me. I'd never do this to anyone. If you can't help me, then it's over. We're thru. I never want to see you again."

And so many other things he said and threats he made... My mind knows it is the Alzheimer's, but my heart doesn't. And, maybe he is right. Maybe, I did fail him. I could have taken better care of him. I should have been more insistent on seeking help sooner. Maybe, I was taking the easy way out when I should have done differently.

The nurse came in with his meds before I left. He was still agitated but not as much. I mentioned to her that his skin seemed clammy and she might want to take a blood glucose reading. It could have been from exertion, but felt more like it did when he was having a hypoglycemic reaction. She brought him juice to drink to bring up the level.

I called the desk at night. At 10 p.m., even after the juice, his blood glucose was down to 33. He was given more juice and ice cream which he refused to eat.

Saturday, June 24, 2006

Last night and this morning I walked through the house looking at all of Jack's paintings and thinking that he may never live in this house again. If his foot or leg is amputated, he will never walk again. The house could be adapted for that. But if he remains so agitated, how could I restrain him from hurting himself?

Went to the hospital at noon. Found that they had moved Jack once again. He needed a sitter so they placed him in a room with another man who needed one. The sitters do precisely that. They stay in the room and make sure the patients are not doing something they are not supposed to be doing. In the case of the other man, he has pneumonia. He has an oxygen tube in his nose which he keeps trying to remove. He's a quiet little guy, the total opposite of the man in the other room.

Jack was fine when I entered the room. He was groggy, but calm. I gave him a kiss and hugged him. I asked the nurses to remove the hand restraints and they did. We talked a little but he was saying things in that very low voice that he has been using recently. I bent over to hear everything he was saying. Most of it was jumbled. The meds were undoubtedly affecting him.

He ate well at lunch, an entire bowl of broth with crackers, a good part of a salisbury steak, fruit, gelatin, ice cream and milk. I was delighted.

All afternoon he dozed off and on. He might have slept if it were quiet. But every noise roused him. Around 3:30 p.m., I told him I was leaving for a little while but I would be back before dinner.

Tricia and I went to 4:30 p.m. Mass. It was so long that we left after Communion. I dropped Tricia off in front of the house and drove straight to the hospital.

Jack was agitated. Where was I? The nurse said that he had gotten rambunctious. Sundowning again. A repeat of last night. Apparently, she had called me at home. (There was a message on the answering machine which I listened to later at night.) Jack insisted that I told him I would only be gone for fifteen minutes. He wasn't angry, only upset.

His dinner tray had come while I was gone. He had only eaten a little bite of the mashed potatoes, none of the appetizing turkey which is a food he has always enjoyed, none of the ice cream and only drank a few ounces of milk.

He began rolling his top sheet up into folds as he pulled it up and away from his legs. He said he had to get out of here. I

THEY LIVED AT OUR HOUSE

gently told him he had to stay until his foot was better. After he folded up the sheet and put it on the side, he began trying to take off the posey. He started working on the side straps and trying to open the latches. Then he attempted wriggling his arms out of the sleeves and got the IV in his left arm tangled in the mesh.

The sitter, a young girl with a fresh face and huge blue eyes, and three nurses and aides watched. They tried distracting him.

"How long have you been married?"

"Forty years." (Correct and interesting that it was right.)

"Where did you meet your wife?"

"Alaska." (Not right.)

He kept saying that he had to get out of here. They watched with fascination as he successfully pulled the strap out of one latch. He wriggled his arms and head out of the posey (he was actually free but didn't recognize it), then turned over and tried unlatching the other side, pulling that strap out. I could see on a few faces that they were amazed. I was not. He had spent his whole life determined to succeed in solving problems and he would never give up until he figured them out. By this time there were seven nurses and aides in the room.

They did nothing, allowing him to struggle with the second strap. Good thinking. But as soon as Jack made a move to get out of bed, they sprang into action. And all hell broke loose. They put the hand restraints back on, undoing one at a time to get his arms into the sleeves of the posey. He fought for his life. Seven people had a difficult time and called for hospital security. They came tearing up like they were after a criminal. But when they reached the room, they were kind. One said, "Remember me?" So they had apparently been called on Thursday night.

There were so many staff in there, I backed out into the hall. I knew Jack wanted my help and I couldn't give it. Seeing me did not diminish his agitation. It increased it. All our life together we have helped each other. Now, when he needed it most, he thought I was failing him.

I know this is what Alzheimer's does, but it is so hard to witness. It kills one's heart to know that there is nothing you can do. Except pray. And that I am constantly doing. O Jesus, take him home where he will be free of all earthly restraints.

The staff was very solicitous of me, as well. I explained that I did understand what was happening and why. But it still hurt because I couldn't help him. He would be horrified to learn that he had acted this way were he in his right mind. He has always been quiet, gentle, dignified. How humiliating for him! I hope that his failing memory retains nothing of these episodes. This is his purgatory.

I did not go back into the hospital room. I did not want to further upset Jack by letting him see me there and not being able to help him. Furtively, I watched from a distance. When he grew calm, I left.

Around 10 p.m., I spoke with the night nurse. She said he had had a hypoglycemic reaction and that was remedied. She said she still wanted to give him the heparin preparatory to the angiogram to be done on Monday and change his adult briefs. I complimented her on the use of that term and told her I wished all the nurses and aides would use it instead of diaper. Adults are relinquishing a lot being in the hospital and adult brief is much less assaulting to their dignity.

She also said she was making recommendations to the doctor regarding using a type of insulin that is injected once a day and avoids the high and low readings. She spoke about Alzheimer's Disease and its effects and all the disorientation that results when a situation is changed. A truth I know well. Her compassionate words were balm for my heart on this night.

Sunday, June 25, 2006

It still seems unreal not to see or hear Jack at home. In forty years of marriage, we have been only apart from each other for two weeks. One week when Jack was hospitalized and one week when I was in the hospital many years ago.

When I arrived at the hospital early this afternoon, Jack was calm. The nurse sat him in a chair by his bed and he was shaved by the room sitter, a pleasant young man who was in the nursing program at Harper College. While he was sitting in the chair, Jack whispered, "Uncle Harry is having surgery. He's not well." (He did have an Uncle Harry.) A while later, he said, "Alice in Wonderland is supposed to come."

Around 4 p.m., his manner changed and again he became obsessed with leaving. More sundowning. He became very angry because I wasn't helping him.

The nurse and I talked about the sundowning. She said it happened all the time with elderly patients, particularly those with significant dementia. It was more difficult for the families than the nurses. Often, it is the first time that family members have encountered it. The nurses see it all the time. I had read about it and had seen evidence of it at home where I did try to keep the environment and schedules the same. It is always more pronounced in the hospital environment where all is unfamiliar.

Once home from the hospital this evening and checking voicemail, there was a message from my brother Frank. His father-in-law had died on Saturday. It was very quick. He was grilling a steak on the patio and a massive heart attack felled him. He managed to crawl into the house where he was found on Sunday. This is a huge loss not only for his children but also for Frank. He was a good man and for the past twenty years Frank had come to regard him as the dad he never had.

Monday, June 26, 2006

The vascular surgeon did the angiogram this morning. Later in the afternoon, he came into the room. He checked the pulse in Jack's leg and let me listen. You could hear the differences by listening to the various areas of the leg. He said the angiogram showed no circulation below the right ankle. If one or two of the arteries was okay, bypass might be possible. It was not possible without any viable blood vessels. The angiogram was shown to me on the computer at the nurses' station.

Because of the worsening mental condition, he opted not to do surgery. He said that the skin on the toe would harden. The gangrene would reoccur. The antibiotic would keep the infection under control. He said that Jack probably doesn't feel much pain because of the severe diabetic sensory nerve impairment and neuropathy.

While we were sitting at the computer, I noticed that in the list of tests under Jack's name was the MRI that had been done last year. I asked the doctor if I could see it. No problem. He brought it up and pointed to all the areas of the brain that showed atrophy and destruction. The devastation was stunning to see, knowing what a normal brain looks like. The areas of atrophy were spread throughout the brain.

We had a long conversation. The surgeon's suggestion was to place Jack in a care facility. It would be too difficult to care for him at home, even with help. There were so many areas where he needed skilled nursing and there was the even greater problem of dealing with the recurring agitation triggered by the Alzheimer's.

Tuesday, June 27, 2006

A quiet day at the hospital. Jack slept all afternoon. I am reluctant to relegate his care to a nursing facility. I spoke with the social worker and some other staff members on the feasibility of bringing Jack home. It is my decision. But I note that they see how much care he is receiving in the hospital and do not think it can be done at home. I called the lawyer to find out what I need to do legally. The appointment is at 3 p.m. on Thursday.

Wednesday, June 28, 2006

My hopes of possibly bringing Jack home came crashing down today. He was so very agitated that I realized fully that he is not improving and I could not take care of him at home. I left the hospital early to do online research of homes in the area. The social worker gave me a list. I spent the evening and a good part of the night online comparing homes and reading inspection reports.

Thursday, June 29, 2006

My younger sister and her husband had come in from out of state to attend the funeral for Frank's father-in-law. They offered to tour the various care facilities with me. I would not have to do it alone. What a blessing!

My first choice was a senior care center close to home. It is a huge complex with all levels of living from independent homes to assisted living to skilled care. Each person has a private room which is good. But the rooms are full of dark wood and seemed depressing. No color. No light.

The second facility we visited is a better choice. The rooms are large and airy. There is a private room available.

After sharing sandwiches, my sister and her husband left to begin the long drive home. Frank came. I had to speak with the case manager at the hospital so they could start the paperwork. I went to visit Jack in his room. Frank was visibly shaken to see him. There were tears in his eyes as we left. He put his arm around me. It felt so good not to be walking the corridors alone.

Then it was on to the appointment with the lawyer. He mentioned a number of things I must do to preserve assets for Tricia's future. There were changes in the trust and other documents, and financial steps that needed to be taken.

Frank and I stopped for a quick dinner. He drove downtown to get some time sensitive work done at the office. I needed to tackle the stacks of paperwork necessary to affect these changes. It was a very long night.

Friday, June 30, 2006

After gathering together the clothes and necessities Jack would need at the rehab facility, I put them in the car. It seemed surreal. As the Alzheimer's had progressed these past few years, I had always wondered what the future held. Then suddenly, a week ago, our little world was turned upside-down. And here I was doing the unthinkable.

The case manager at the hospital called and said they were moving Jack at 1 p.m. I went on ahead to the rehab facility and put his clothes and other items in the room. Then I sat down with the placement director to fill out a seemingly unending stream of forms. As I was still filling out the forms, I saw the ambulance attendants wheeling Jack into the facility. He looked so still and fragile.

One of the forms pertained to the patient's primary care physician, an internist, not a specialist. Jack does not have one. The endocrinologist, a specialist, is his only physician. On the rare occasions when Jack has had a cold or flu, he would call the endocrinologist, who would prescribe an antibiotic or other medicines needed and Jack would recover. The placement director informed me that it was mandatory in care facilities to have a primary care physician. The facility had two doctors who cared for the patients there. With my approval, she would assign Jack to one of them.

At first, Jack was quiet in his room. Therapists came in and spoke with me about his decline. They were astonished to learn that he was so independent just one week ago.

As the afternoon wore on, he became more agitated. The nursing facility does not use restraints which is good. The bed is low. Mats can be placed on the floor so that if he did get out of bed when he shouldn't, he wouldn't injure himself. What they do use is an alert monitor. One end is hooked onto the patient's clothing. The other end is hooked onto the mattress. If the patient tries to get out of bed, the cord is pulled out of the base which then emits a loud warning to the staff.

Stroking his hand helped Jack to grow calm and to rest contentedly in bed. At one point, as I stood by the side of the bed, he looked over my shoulder and said, "Isn't that nice. Betty came to see me." (His oldest sister who had died fifteen years ago.)

Saturday, July 1, 2006

When I arrived at the rehab facility, Jack was dressed in a shirt and pants and was sitting in a wheelchair in the dining room. He wouldn't touch any of his lunch. He would mumble, "You eat it." The aide said he ate all of his breakfast.

Afterward the nurse settled him in the common area near the desk and I sat in a chair next to him. He became fixated on the leg pad on the wheelchair and kept picking at it. While we were sitting there, Tricia called the nurses' station. I walked over to answer the phone. I just started talking with her when I heard a loud crash behind me. Jack had bent so far over, he fell on the floor wheelchair and all. He had a bump on his head and ice was put on it. X-rays were taken as a precaution.

At that time the internist came down the hall. He spoke with me about Jack's condition and examined him. He concurred that the situation was a Catch 22.

About three, I left Jack settled in bed and somewhat calm. Tricia and I went to 4:30 p.m. Mass. A couple we see at Mass each weekend asked where Jack was and we explained the situation. They were saddened.

This evening was spent on the phone letting everyone know that Jack was in a rehab center. They all assured me that he is in their prayers. In truth, praying for him is the best thing that they can do for him now. He is definitely in God's hands. The future is a total unknown. I can only take it one day at a time. Each day is difficult enough on its own without trying to add the worry of days to come.

Sunday, July 2, 2006

The rehab center called in the morning to say Jack had gotten out of bed and fallen. He was okay. The mats were on the floor so they cushioned his fall.

When I walked into Jack's room after noon, he was in bed. He seemed a little more alert and quiet. He was dressed and shaved. He slept some. When he awoke, he started to work on the railing at the upper sides of the bed.

One of the most unusual phenomena has been the hand movements that Jack started making in the hospital. They have increased since he has been at the rehab center. The movements are slow and gentle. He will reach up as though he is trying to touch an invisible something. Or to the side. Or even toward the ground. Always the movements are graceful. His hand reaches out toward the spot where his eyes are looking. But his eyes do not focus. He lives in his own little world.

How I wonder what he is seeing or hoping to touch or is touching? These episodes are astonishing to see and I treasure them.

Monday, July 3, 2006

This morning I went to the 9 a.m. weekday Mass for the first time. It truly is food for my soul to hear the familiar words and receive the Eucharist. Even though my head is spinning and I feel like I couldn't think my way out of a paper bag, I feel a certain undefinable peace. I need to attend Mass every morning.

Physically, I have been walking this road alone for the past two weeks. Emotionally and spiritually, I feel so empty. I need God's help and grace.

Through Father Kane, who was celebrant of the Mass this morning, God gave me a sign that He is by my side. For over twenty years I have been trying to find the words to one of the responses that was used after the consecration many years ago. All I could remember was the ending "...He is joy for all ages" which I have dearly loved all these years. I love the idea of Jesus being joy for all ages, whether of people and children, or of all the years gone by and to come. I have looked in every missal and book I came across to no avail. My mind was elsewhere and I was half listening when I heard the words, "He is joy for all ages." Father Kane had recited my prayer!

After Mass, I went up to the woman who had given the readings. She did not know the prayer by heart and looked in the sacramentary. It was not there. She looked in the missal. She could not find it. She suggested that I ask Father Kane.

I went to the sacristy and asked him if he could write the words down for me. He obliged. At last I have the prayer that has eluded me for twenty years.

> *Keep in mind that Jesus Christ has died for us*
> *And is risen from the dead.*
> *He is our saving Lord.*
> *He is Joy for all ages.*

For me this is a sign that confirms my desire to attend daily Mass now that I am able to do so.

Per the lawyer's recommendations I cashed in a certificate of deposit and opened an account in my name with Frank as co-owner. The banks were busy and I had a late start to the rehab center. I didn't arrive until mid afternoon.

I stopped at the nurses' desk and was immediately asked what Jack did for a living. I replied that he had been a graphic artist for thirty-five years. The nurse said that earlier in the day he had asked her, "Who is the art director here?" She said he had eaten his breakfast and was in the hall for a while. He had made a thousand attempts to get up. He was given a newspaper, then a magazine.

When I entered his room, Jack knew I was there but didn't say anything. He no longer responds in the usual way of greeting another. He was in his little world, half snoozing, half awake and engrossed in pulling or pushing or picking at something.

At one point I was holding his hand. He took his other hand and began moving it up my arm toward my sleeve. He slipped his fingers under the edge of the short sleeve and began pushing it up toward the shoulder. It was very gentle and mesmerized him for at least half an hour. I stood by the bed, bent over the railing stroking his hair or shoulder. All was peaceful, calm.

Suddenly, the mood changed (again the sundowning!) and he became restless, pulling the sheet out from the foot of the bed and trying to dismantle the bed rails. The nurse came in and gave him his meds hidden in applesauce. After a while he grew calm. With the help of an aide, I sat him in a wheelchair. We worked our way to the dining room. He was calm enough to respond when I asked him to eat. He ate mashed potatoes and drank milk.

Afterward, he was content enough to sit by the nurses' desk. He allowed me to give him a kiss before I left.

Tuesday, July 4, 2006

Awoke early and went to morning Mass. Spoke with Father Pat who asked about Jack. I told him briefly what the situation was. I asked him if the priest who offers Mass at the rehab center would do an Anointing of the Sick if I called and requested it. Father Pat said he himself would be happy to do it.

Tricia is dog sitting all this week at the home of the dog owners. It is a 24/7 job so she will not be home until Sunday. She has not seen her dad since I drove him to the hospital almost two weeks ago. There has been such a deterioration in look and personality and I am not sure that she will understand why. She has never seen the level of agitation that has occurred in the hospital and I know it would frighten her. Since I have no idea when it will occur, I have not asked her to come with me to the hospital or now to the rehab center and she has not asked if she can see him. We talk about him all the time and the problem with his foot. She continues to pray for him and is content to do that as her way of helping.

Stopped at a big box store on my way to the rehab center to get pants with elastic waists for Jack. All his life he would only wear long pants which require belts and are useless in a nursing center. It's summer and the store does not have any long pants with elastic, only shorts.

Throughout the afternoon Jack slept off and on. The nurse noticed that his stomach was distended. She used a catheter to remove 700 cc of fluid.

Around 4 p.m., the agitation surfaced as sundowning kicked in again. Jack grew calmer at dinnertime. He kept staring out the dining room window and trying to say something. But it was so quiet and jumbled I couldn't understand what he wanted to say. He ate part of a grilled cheese sandwich and drank the milk. He was calm when I wheeled him back to his room.

But once we were in the room, he wanted me to wheel him out the door. When I told him I could not do that, he told me how useless I was and how I had let him down. It was a very bad scene. He didn't want to stay in the chair. The nurse noticed his restlessness and readied him for bed. He was lying with his eyes closed when I left. One thing I did notice today was the absence of those delicate hand movements.

Never have I felt so depressed and deflated as I did on the drive home. My head hurt. My heart hurt. I was failing my Jack, being unable to have him with me at home. Unable to do much for him at all. How I wish I could!

When I arrived home, there was a message on the phone from my dear next door neighbor. "Come on over. The family is having a late dinner and we won't take 'no' for an answer." The shish-ka-bobs, rice, salad and fruit were delicious. But the best part was seeing her grandchildren, the youngest only three weeks old. That was food for the soul and balm for the heart. What a thoughtful, precious neighbor she is.

Wednesday, July 5, 2006
One of my sisters who lives in Indiana called insisting that I needed a day of respite from two weeks of hospitals and rehab centers. She and her husband drove out. We went to lunch and to an outlet store that she wanted to see. As we looked around the shop, I noticed how much difficulty she is having in walking. It was a muggy day which also made breathing more difficult for her. She was sacrificing her comfort to comfort me.

When we returned home, we sat on the patio for a long time savoring dessert. It was a perfect day. And I am grateful for my sister's thoughtfulness, even though I kept wondering how Jack is doing. No phone calls - a good sign.

Thursday, July 6, 2006
This morning at Mass, I was thinking about how the strong Heavey constitution is a detriment to Jack. There is no reversal of this situation without a miracle. I am not asking for one. All I want for him is freedom from pain and suffering and humiliation and all of earth's restraints.

Today, Jack was dressed but lying in bed. Unfocused. A few hand movements. Whispering quietly. The therapist came to take Jack for his session. He had to sit him up. Jack sat slumped over on the edge of the bed with the therapist's arm and hand behind him. When the therapist purposely removed his arm, Jack started to fall back. It was a very short therapy session. He could not stand for any length of time.

The therapists have been amazed to learn that Jack actually walked into the hospital on his own just two weeks ago. They find the rate of decline astonishing. In some ways, it does not surprise me. Knowing Jack, I believe that he has been drawing on every ounce of his reserve energy to do as much as he could every day to retain his independence. He has little energy left.

Friday, July 7, 2006

The care coordinator is worried about Jack's blood glucose readings. They are all over the place, with one being as high as five hundred. The doctor is upping the insulin. He is not eating. Where is the glucose coming from? The diabetes is not good for the foot. The foot infection is not good for the diabetes.

All of the diseases are working against Jack. If he only had Alzheimer's, that would be bad enough. If he only had the foot problem, that would be bad enough. The combination with the long-standing diabetes and infection is overwhelming. Without saying it, she is trying to prepare me for the inevitable.

Jack's only focus now is on himself. It is the only reality he knows. He is very attentive to how different parts of his body feel. He fiddles with his clothes and covers. When he awoke, he tried covering his face with the sheet. Then he began to reach out once more for the objects in the air that only he can see. Those graceful movements of hand and arm.

Saturday, July 8, 2006

I only spent a few hours with Jack today. He was sleeping off and on. His sleep was not calm, but rather disturbed.

Picked up Tricia and we went to 4:30 p.m. Mass. Then I drove her back to the house where she is still dog sitting. I was drained when I came home and once again ignored the mountain of paperwork on my desk. Nothing matters. Only Jack.

Sunday, July 9, 2006

I felt better this morning and attended to the necessary paperwork before going to see Jack. He was clean shaven and sleeping placidly, not disturbed as yesterday. Such sleep is the best thing for him. Left after an hour or so.

Monday, July 10, 2006

After morning Mass, I finished the paperwork and made an appointment with the lawyer for Friday. Left for the rehab center around lunch. Jack's tray was in his room. He was very lethargic and was slumped in the bed. He didn't fiddle very much with his clothing or anything else. He did not respond when I tried to feed him lunch. He just slept. I gathered up his wash and left around 3 p.m.

Tricia and I had errands and we stopped for a quick dinner. Afterward, we took a walk around the neighborhood and then sat on the patio for a while. There was a slight breeze and the air was refreshing and relaxing.

When we entered the house, there were two messages on the answering machine. One was from the rehab center saying they had done some blood work on Jack and the results were not good. They were transporting him to the hospital. The message was sent at 6:30 p.m. It was already 8 p.m. I was kicking myself for not checking for messages after we returned from our walk, rather than going directly out back. I called the nurses' station at the rehab center. She said that the transport was late and had actually just arrived.

I called a cab since I did not know when I would be coming home or in what condition.

Jack was lying on a gurney in cubicle twelve. He was not responsive. His legs were bent to the side and looked bonier than usual. A nurse had just started an IV and blood was being drawn. The fluids made him more responsive. He began to fidget with the IV leads. I was told he was dehydrated, had an electrolyte imbalance and was in renal failure.

The ER doctor asked questions about his past history, the first hospitalization two weeks ago, the rehab center, and the dementia. She related that her father also had had Alzheimer's Disease. When he needed to be hospitalized, he, too, experienced the same decline. The family even had a feeding tube inserted, but later removed it. She said it was a common occurrence in patients with long-term Alzheimer's Disease. They experienced a significant decline when transferred from home (familiar) to hospital (foreign).

As I stood in the cubicle stroking Jack's hair and his thin shoulders, I could hear the nurse at the desk across the way giving Jack's vital stats to CCU. She said the renal failure was so acute, there was a question of whether he would pull out of it.

The Critical Care Unit is divided into three pods, each with twelve rooms around the perimeter of a central nurses' core. Everything is wide open and inviting. State of the art beds with the ability to handle all diverse critical care needs. The rooms are approximately seventeen square feet with polished wood floors, serene walls and furnishings. What a difference from the regular hospital rooms with their overly cramped conditions, especially the ones with double beds.

The nephrologist spoke with me and said the BUN was 199, one of the highest she had ever seen. They would do dialysis, if I would agree to it. She was not sure how effective it would be. I signed the release form to allow it. I stayed with Jack until the dialysis was given.

I called Tricia and told her that her dad was okay. I would spend the night and keep her informed. While the nurses were caring for Jack, I would stand in the empty family lounge alone staring out into the darkness. Not only the darkness of the night, but also the darkness of the immediate future. Watched a gray dawn break gradually.

Tuesday, July 11, 2006

Around 6 a.m. I called Frank to let him know that Jack was back in the hospital in the critical care unit.

By 11 a.m., Jack was looking much better and was resting without too much agitation. The pristine openness of the CCU and his being neatly tucked in prompted me to think that it would be a good time for Tricia to see her dad. She had not seen him since we first drove to the hospital on June 22nd. There was never a time when I wanted her to see him in the condition he was in. It would have been too traumatic for her.

When I arrived home, I asked her if she wanted to go. She was eager. On the way to the hospital, I explained that her dad had changed. He couldn't really talk and his eyes would not focus on her.

When we reached his room, she started to walk thru the glass door, took one look at her dad, and burst into tears. "That's not my Daddy!" She ran out of the room and down the corridor. She was sobbing uncontrollably. I followed and put my arms around her trembling shoulders. We just stood for a few minutes with her wrapped in my arms. Then she composed herself and said she would be okay. I suggested she go to the family lounge and wait for me.

I returned to the CCU where the physician/director was waiting to speak with me. He suggested that hospice might be the best thing for Jack. He said the attending physician was not in agreement. I would need to speak with him, if I decided that hospice was best. The attending physician would have to concur or sign off the case.

As I was talking with the director, out of the corner of my eye I saw Tricia walk back into her dad's room and sit down. She stayed with him for the rest of the day. He was somewhat agitated and definitely in his own little world, reaching out with his hands for those invisible (to us) objects.

When the nurses did records and the floor was closed, we went down to the Oasis Cafeteria for a bit of dinner. Returning to the floor, I met with the liaison from hospice who explained the program. It sounded very peaceful and comforting and all encompassing. Hospice looks after all the needs - physical, spiritual, emotional - of the patient as well as the family.

The nurses were finally able to connect via phone with the attending physician who said to me:

"I can't believe you are considering this. His problems are manageable. First, we need to do more dialysis to get the kidneys back to a manageable level. When that is stabilized, then we need to address the problem of his not eating and dehydration. We can use a naso-gastric tube and eventually a permanent abdominal one. You can push all the nutrients and hydration you need and bring the body to a normal level. When that is done, then we can amputate the leg at a point where there is viable tissue so that it will heal.

"The Alzheimer's can be taken care of by the neurologist and psychiatrist. He can live for several years. No point in giving up unless nature takes it course. We can correct these things and he can go back to the rehab center.

"It's too early for hospice. He can be improved with a feeding tube. Hospice pushes a lot of painkillers. I would not go in that direction. We should keep on doing what we are doing.

"Think about it. This is not liver cancer. I'll do whatever you tell me to do. But if you push for hospice, the patient expires. At this level, I am not convinced he needs that."

I was totally distraught after that monologue. One of the young nurses with very deep dark eyes consoled me. She offered me as much advice as she could without overstepping the boundaries of her profession. She gave me a hug I desperately needed.

While I was on the phone with the internist, Tricia waited in the family room. On the way home, she said to me, "I'm glad that I saw Daddy. But I don't know if I want to come tomorrow."

I told her that was perfectly okay. She should do only what she was comfortable doing. She said, "I wish Daddy would go to sleep and God would take him and he wouldn't have to suffer anymore." I told her it was the perfect prayer.

My mind was in turmoil. How do you decide another person's life? At home, I read the entire packet of information regarding hospice. Could I bring Jack home with hospice? What would seeing her dad die do to Tricia? What would it be like? Would he be deprived of food and water? Would he starve?

I went online to learn what the Church's position was on feeding tubes. Were they ordinary means of treatment? Was I wrong if I refused the use of a tube or dialysis?

It was a night from hell. My mind was racing so much, it was difficult to fall asleep. If I did, I would awaken in a short while. The realization of this decision that I had to make would descend on my chest with a heaviness too crushing to bear. To continue treatment or not? To grasp for life or say enough is enough? To decide another person's fate? It is not supposed to be this way. It is supposed to be God's decision, not mine. I am not qualified to do His work.

Wednesday, July 12, 2006

Since I couldn't sleep, I went early to pray in the Perpetual Adoration Chapel at our church. My heart was as heavy as ever as I knelt there with my mind spinning. All my muddled brain could draw on was the prayer that had saved me many times in the past.

Trust Him when dark doubts assail you.
Trust Him when your strength is small.
Trust Him when to simply trust Him
Seems the hardest thing of all.

And then in my mind, I heard a voice say, "Put it all in My Hands. Be at peace." The heaviness in my heart lifted. I walked out of the chapel feeling calm even though I still had the decision to make.

I had hoped to speak with Father Pat but he was not there. He was doing a funeral Mass later in the morning. Father Denis was celebrating the morning Mass. As he walked into the chapel, he announced the hymn to be sung, *Morning Has Broken*. Providence was reassuring me with this favorite hymn of mine which is rarely sung in recent years.

After Mass, Father Denis was alone in the sacristy removing his vestments when I walked in and asked him if he had a few minutes. He readily said, "Yes."

I explained the situation to him briefly. He asked, "What would your husband want?"

I replied, "I know that if Jack did not have Alzheimer's, he would have had the amputation and worked hard to master a prosthesis. But he would not want to live in the conditions proposed."

He told me that when he was chaplain at St. Alexius Hospital (news to me) he worked with families whose doctors wanted to try all sorts of procedures. For these few doctors it is a profitable business but it caused much grief for the families.

He said that if hospice had been offered, accept it eagerly. It is a very Christian organization whose members do not starve patients or allow dehydration or assist them in ending their lives. Hospice professionals focus on comfort care and are concerned not only about the patient, but also about the whole family, on all levels - physically, emotionally, psychologically and spiritually.

He asked if Jack had had the Anointing of the Sick. I answered that to my knowledge I did not think so. He asked me to check with the chaplain at the hospital to see if he had done so. If not, I should call him in the afternoon and he would come.

The hospice nurse, called shortly after I came home and set up an appointment for 12:30 p.m. I hurried over to the hospital. Jack was the calmest I had ever seen him in three weeks. Since the night before he had not been given any medications except for pain relief.

We spent almost two hours reviewing Jack's clinical report written after his admission to CCU early Tuesday. There was one disturbing entry indicating that there was some minor tissue necrotization occurring in other parts of the body. I did not know this. It explained why Jack was so fixated on one or another area when agitated. This was a recent occurrence and definitely not a good sign.

We discussed the hospice organization and I signed the necessary papers. One very thorny problem was the attending physician. The hospice nurse decided that she and the CCU nurses would find another physician who would be willing to take over. Afterward I would phone the internist, advise him of my decision and inform him that another physician would attend to Jack.

There was no record of anointing by the chaplain. I left a message for Father Denis asking him to come, if available.

I returned to Jack. He was still calm. He tried to tell me something but he couldn't form the words and his voice was almost inaudible. As with all good plans of mice and men, about ten minutes later the internist walked into the room. Since I had only met him once, he said,

"You probably don't remember me."

"Oh, yes, I do."

He promptly walked over to the bed and began addressing Jack and asking the nurse all sorts of questions. He checked

Jack's heart with his stethoscope and did the usual perfunctory actions. When he was finished, he turned around and said, "I see on the chart that you are going with hospice."

"Doctor, it is a difficult decision, but I favor hospice as being in Jack's best interest. It is what he would want."

"I think you are making a mistake. He's not ready for that. There are things we could do. We can do dialysis, we can use a feeding tube, we can do an amputation on the leg where there is a good blood supply for healing, we can use medicines for the dementia and psychosis. If it were my decision, I would not let emotions interfere."

"Doctor, I am not making this decision on an emotional level."

"Think about it."

At that moment, the young nurse, who had been standing by quietly, said, "Doctor, before you go, there is something you should see." She walked over to Jack's bed and he followed. She showed him the other sites of necrotization. He observed, then turned around and said,

"Perhaps you have made the right decision."

I thanked him for his services and extended my hand. He shook it and left.

The nurse said, "How would he like to live with multiple amputations?"

Later the head nurse came in all smiles. "I heard about your encounter with the internist." She and all the staff in CCU felt vindicated in their opposition to his proposals. She gave me the name of the physician who would attend Jack in hospice. The name sounded familiar.

Shortly thereafter, Father Denis arrived. He spoke to Jack who tried to respond but couldn't. Father Denis prayed over him for the forgiveness of his sins and gave him absolution. He asked Jack if he knew who he was. Jack nodded. He asked Jack if he knew Who he would be receiving in the Eucharist. I could see the recognition in his face. Father Denis held up the host, then broke off a small piece and put it on Jack's tongue. The nurse gave him a sip of water to help him swallow it. Then Father Denis anointed his forehead and his hands with the oil of the sick. Jack was spiritually ready to begin his journey Home. Joy and peace flooded my soul.

After Father Denis left, the nurse commented on how dry Jack's mouth was. She'd been using special swabs all day to keep it moist. She wanted to give him something to eat or drink. I suggested his beloved vanilla ice cream. She immediately set off to get a cup. Jack ate every spoonful she gave him. He even gave her a little smile which pleased her. She's very young, a true nurse with a compassionate heart.

It was good to be able to touch Jack and get a little kiss from him. He'd pucker his lips if I asked him for a kiss. For the most part I have been unable to give him any of the physical contact I had hoped to give him because of the agitation. That has been the hardest part of this whole ordeal. All I have wanted to do was to put my arms around him and hold him close, or even just hold his hand or stroke his hair as I have always done. Mostly, I've been rebuffed, not by Jack because he doesn't know what he is doing, but by the disease that has claimed his mind and thus governs his actions. It gives me a little glimpse of the pain Mary endured knowing that she could not comfort her Son, Jesus, during His suffering.

Plans are in the works to move Jack to hospice on the ninth floor this evening. As I was waiting for the elevator, I met the nurse who gave me a hug yesterday. She was happy to learn that Jack was going to hospice.

Thursday, July 13, 2006

After morning Mass, I went directly to the hospital. Jack had been moved to the ninth floor late yesterday evening. I was hoping to speak to the physician who would now be attending to Jack. My hope was that he would still be there. He was not. He called up to the floor and I spoke with him by phone at the nurse's station. I stressed the fact that Jack was more agitated than he had been on Wednesday. He said they were giving him morphine every four hours but that can create peaks and valleys. He would order an IV infusion so that a steady amount would be going into the bloodstream at all times. He said that either he or his colleague would monitor it over the weekend and adjust it accordingly.

Because I knew the name was familiar, at the end of the conversation I asked him if other family members were also in the medical profession. He said his grandfather had had an office in Oak Park. I related to him that it was his grandfather who had initially diagnosed Jack's diabetes forty-two years ago. He said he would tell his grandmother because she always loved to hear stories about patients that he meets who were also treated by his grandfather. Life coming full circle.

Jack was not as calm as yesterday. He did allow me to kiss him but he did not pucker up. He tried to speak, but it was inaudible. He was feeling pain which made him very restless. His mouth was dry. I tried giving him a little of his much loved ice cream to moisten it. He was eager to take it, opening his mouth when I asked. But he couldn't swallow it today. There is a decided decline from yesterday.

In early afternoon, the hospice caregivers came and did a compassionate job of bathing his body. They even had a cap with shampoo in it that cleans the oil out of the hair without the need for rinsing. They were very efficient, but tender. It was very painful for Jack at times when he was moved.

I held his hands while he was being washed. How my heart aches for him! I can only hope that all the suffering has earned him heaven as I have been praying for so long. It is my only consolation. I truly believe that all victims of Alzheimer's have their purgatory here on earth and do go straight to the joy and peace and glory of heaven.

The nurse set up the morphine infusion. Shortly after it was begun, Jack gradually relaxed and fell into a deep sleep. How good it was not to see him suffering. I was praying the rosary. The hospice social worker knocked on the door. She walked into the room and suggested that since Jack was sleeping peacefully, I should get a change of scene. We walked down the hall to the family lounge.

She started talking and asking about Jack. Fifteen minutes later, the hospice chaplain joined us. They spent about two hours with me, mostly letting me talk, answering the questions I had and allaying any concerns. I voiced the most important question I had, "How do you know when death is imminent?" The chaplain gave me a thin pamphlet to read later.

What a marvelous pamphlet! I read it as soon as I returned to Jack's room as he was still asleep. It describes the signs and symptoms of the dying process. As I read them, I realized that many of these had been occurring in Jack during the past few months. But I didn't know them for what they were. It is comforting to know that the process has been occurring for a long time, not just in the past three weeks. On the other hand, if I had known, perhaps I would have considered hospice earlier and saved Jack the agony of the past week.

After finishing the booklet, I stood by Jack's bed and held his hand while he slept. I told Jack that he could go. I didn't want him to suffer another second. And I told his mom that I knew how eager she was to have her son with her again - her pride and joy. Whenever God was ready, Jack was hers. Jack was asleep when I left at 6:30 p.m. It was so good to be able to bend down and kiss him. The times he would let me do that in the past three weeks have been so few.

About 9:20 p.m., the night nurse called and said that Jack's breathing was labored and I might want to come. I called Tricia who was out with a friend. I told her I would take a cab to the hospital. Her friend said she would come by and drive me there. She did.

When I arrived on the ninth floor, I walked directly down the quiet corridor to Jack's room. The nurse stopped me just as I reached the door. She said she was sorry. After calling me she went back to Jack's room and he was gone. And that's how it ended. Forty years together.

I walked into the room and the nurse closed the door. Jack's mouth was very slightly open. His skin was cool to the touch. I cried. I prayed. I touched. I kissed. And I thanked God. Jack was at peace at last. No more humiliation and confusion and pain. Only joy and peace and love.

After twenty minutes, there was a knock on the door and the hospital chaplain entered. He hugged me. We spoke about Jack. His mom has Alzheimer's, so he knows. We prayed. The hospice nurse came in to make the official determination of death. The chaplain said that if I called the funeral chapel now, they would come directly to the floor for Jack. If I waited until morning, he would be taken down to the morgue. I did not want that.

The chaplain stayed with me while I went to the family lounge and called the funeral chapel. They said they would come directly to the floor. They arranged for the transference and made an appointment for me to meet with them tomorrow to plan the funeral. I called my brother. He had just readied for bed, but said he would dress, throw a few things in a bag and be on his way. I told him to take his time. I needed to pick up Tricia. I called a cab.

The chaplain accompanied me down to the emergency room entrance to wait with me for the cab. He was paged. He was very reluctant to leave. I said he was needed elsewhere. He hesitated to go. I was alone. Someone else needed him more now. Go.

I sat waiting for the cab and thinking that that was how the last three weeks had mostly been. Alone. Alone walking hospital corridors. Alone dealing with all the complexities of Jack's care. Alone driving back and forth to the rehab center. Alone signing stacks of forms each time a change occurred. Alone in making decisions for his very life. Yet, I truly believe that this was part of my road to Calvary and it can only be walked alone. Also, in truth, when I felt alone, it was only because my eyes couldn't see Him by my side.

These past three weeks had been Jack's crucifixion on the cross of Alzheimer's and bodily deterioration. His torment was over. Joy was now his.

I gave the cabdriver directions to the home of Tricia's friend. The night was sultry and the cabdriver had the windows open. You could smell the heady scent of the flowers and the trees in the air. A creamy gibbous moon, shaded by a thin haze, hung low over the earth. As we drove up Roselle Road, my eyes welled up. There was the building in which Jack had worked for so many years. I had never thought about driving by it when I gave the directions. Of all nights to pass it by. We never drove by it. Yet tonight...

When Tricia slid into the cab, she asked, "How is Daddy?"

I answered, "Fine." It was not a lie. In truth, he is more than fine.

Once inside the house, I told Tricia that her prayers were answered. She understood and cried. We hugged. Then she said, "Now it is just the two of us." And the realization that Jack would never be in this house again hit home.

Friday, July 14, 2006

The morning was damp and drizzly with a humidity and temperature imbalance that caused everything made of glass to steam up. The day was a whirlwind of appointments. The funeral chapel, the church, the appointment I had made with the lawyer, now with a different agenda, the rehab center to retrieve Jack's belongings, home to select clothing for the wake and back to the funeral chapel to deliver it.

At one point, Frank and I stopped to have a quick sandwich. Tricia called to give me some information. Later at night she said to me, "Mom, do you know what you said to me when you were at the restaurant? You said, 'Daddy and I are having lunch.'"

The evening was filled with nonstop phone calls, neighbors thoughtfully dropping by, and Mike dropping off the countertop for the powder room.

At bedtime, Tricia asked, "Mom, do you think Daddy still knows I love him?"

"More than ever because now he can see clearly."

"Do you think he's mad because I prayed that God would take him?"

"No. He is happy with God. Someday, we will be there with him, together again."

Saturday, July 15, 2006

Rest is just an illusion. Thoughts and emotions are running rampant like rivers overflowing their banks and flooding my heart with grief. An early morning walk did nothing to quell the tempest. All around the neighborhood people are pulling weeds, cutting grass, watering flower beds, walking dogs, loading SUVs with paraphernalia for a trip, a picnic or day at the beach. Totally oblivious. I wanted to stand on a corner and scream, "Don't you know what just happened? Don't you know my life has just been turned around one hundred eighty degrees? Don't you know I just lost the love of my life?!"

Back home, as I sat at the kitchen table nibbling toast I really didn't want, my mind could only focus on how quiet and unassuming Jack was. From the depths of grief, a thought arose. Jack will be forgotten! Who will remember Jack? What do our neighbors and friends really know about him? He was never one

THEY LIVED AT OUR HOUSE

to toot his own horn. From somewhere deep inside, a eulogy began to form and I scribbled the words down. Within a half hour, I had written what needed to be said. Now everyone will truly know my Jack.

◊◊◊◊◊◊◊◊◊◊

THEY LIVED AT OUR HOUSE

Who was Jack?

He was the quintessential Irish Quiet Man, who didn't shout from the rooftops when he was happy or scream in indignation when he was beset with trials or grief.

He was the only son – his father's pride, his mother's joy.

He was his sisters' baby brother – who could be a thorn in the side as a boy – but a rock to lean on as a man.

He was the 1940's altar boy who carried his religious convictions into the twenty-first century.

He was the student who took detention for missed homework without explaining that it was the night his mom almost died in an auto accident.

He was the corner prairie athlete who considered being a baseball player.

He was the soldier on the front lines in Korea who fought to preserve freedom for all people.

He was the artist who saw the order and function in the beauties of nature and permeated his life's work with it.

He was the avid fisherman who charted the good spots of many a lake with his dad.

He was the storyteller who always regaled family and friends with countless tales and anecdotes and humorous stories in a quiet, unassuming way.

He was the beloved husband who made his wife's life a joy for forty years.

He was the puffed up, chest proud daddy of his St. Patrick's Day baby and cherished her butterfly kisses.

He was the family man who always put their needs before his own interests.

He was the 'Jack' of all trades who solved every household fix-it problem with ingenuity and determination.

He was the warrior who successfully fought off the ravages of diabetes for four decades.

He was the unsuspecting victim of Alzheimers, as silent as he, stealing the mind of a quiet man, piece by piece.

He was only one of a million people who passed from this world into eternity on July 13, 2006.

He was a quiet, unassuming man who never sought to make waves or stand out in a crowd.

But as the prophet learned, the voice of God is found not in thunder and roaring seas but in a whisper – the quiet voice of a quiet man.

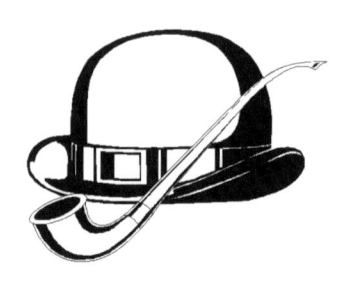

EPILOGUE

Does life go on after Alzheimer's? Yes, it does. Perhaps not always easily, but it does.

Those first few days were a blur of necessary activity. It was real. It was surreal. Even when one knows that these days will come, nothing you have thought prepares you for them. Mundane activities are viewed with a whole new perspective. The whole world dances around you, people driving, shopping, working, playing, seemingly oblivious to the dramatic change in your life.

And with the change are feelings, both bitter and sweet. In the height of the totally draining days caring for a loved one with Alzheimer's, one cannot imagine a day without the worry and stress and agitation. Then, suddenly, it is here. And there are mixed emotions. The realization that no matter how profoundly affected by the disease the person was, he or she was still your loved one and you will never see him or her again. The gratitude that their days of suffering and humiliation and fear are over. They are at peace. The thoughts that perhaps you could have done more or better or been more patient or more loving. The strangeness of days no longer focused on one person. And even stranger, being the focus of other people's attention.

During those first few days and weeks, family, friends, neighbors and the members of our church wrapped their arms around Tricia and me enfolding us in compassion, support and love. Attending grief support sessions and focusing not only on my loss, but also on the devastating losses of other parishioners, helped me walk through the fog of grief and begin to see that life goes on, just new and different. From the shattered clay of the life I had lived with Jack, a new life needed to be created and shaped.

When the grief support sessions ended, three of us who were widowed were loathe to go our separate ways and decided to continue meeting each week. Not to have a perpetual pity party, but to love and laugh and pray and encourage and support each other as we began this walk into the unknown. Immediately two other women joined us. Several have gone on to be with the loves of their life. Other widows come, some who are newly grief stricken and hurting, a few who lost their loves years ago. Within months of losing Jack, LaVerne was moved to a compassionate facility where she lived in loving and secure care until she, too, succumbed to Alzheimer's five years after Jack.

Time has soothed the overwhelming grief that swept over me initially. Every minute of every day is no longer permeated with thoughts of Jack. Have I forgotten about him? No. Do I wish he were still here. Definitely. If I could bring him back, would I? In a heartbeat, but only if he were the Jack with the clear mind and gentle disposition and loving ways.

Never would I want him to endure what he did for another moment. For me, the hardest part of Alzheimer's was not the caregiving. That was only a challenge. Could I make each day as smooth and uneventful as possible? The hardest part was seeing the total destruction of Jack, his personality, his capabilities, his mind. Each loss tore at my heart and left a scar that will always be there as long as I live.

If each of us is given a vial of tears to cry over a loved one, the one I was given was half spent by July 2006. Every time Jack lost an ability, tears flowed. Every time the disease frustrated or humiliated him, tears flowed. Every time his future grew darker, tears flowed.

There are still a few tears left in the vial. At the oddest times, a sound, an object, a thought will trigger a few more tears. Glory shines in these tears as the light catches the prisms in their wetness and creates the most dazzling rainbows in my mind.

These rainbows soothe my heart. In them, I see my Jack eternally happy, free of pain and anxiety, filled with joy, peace and endless love. My prayers have been answered. What more could I ask?

NOTES

1. *The Scarlet Letter.* Nathaniel Hawthorne.
2. *The Notebook.* © Nicholas Sparks.
3. *Into the Shadows.* © Robert DeHaan
4. *A Long Goodnight.* © Daphne Simpkin

ABOUT THE AUTHOR

Stephanie Heavey is a native Chicagoan who resides in the suburbs. Her early career was spent in medical publishing and business. For many years, she designed and produced international costumes for the vastly popular 18-inch dolls. She has been active in Alzheimer's support, funeral ministry and grief support.

Made in the USA
Columbia, SC
27 July 2019